D1797613

Paediatric MCQ Revision for MRCP and MRCPCH

Jane Lucas BM MRCP(UK) DA
Specialist Registrar, Department of Child Health, Loddon
NHS Trust, North Hampshire Hospital, Basingstoke

James Nicholson MA MB BChir MRCP(UK)
Clinical Research Fellow/Honorary Senior Registrar,
Department of Child Health, Southampton General Hospital

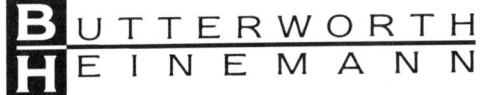

BUTTERWORTH
HEINEMANN

Butterworth-Heinemann
Linacre House, Jordan Hill, Oxford OX2 8DP
A division of Reed Educational and Professional Publishing Ltd

 A member of the Reed Elsevier plc group

OXFORD   BOSTON   JOHANNESBURG
MELBOURNE   NEW DELHI   SINGAPORE

First published 1997

© Reed Educational and Professional Publishing Ltd 1997

British Library Cataloguing in Publication Data
A catalogue record for this book is available from the British Library

ISBN 0 7506 3014 0

Composition by Scribe Design, Gillingham, Kent
Printed and bound in Great Britain by Biddles Ltd,
Guildford and King's Lynn

To Carolyn and Chris

Contents

Preface

Success in the MRCP examination is a requirement for admission to the Royal College of Paediatrics and Child Health, and to the Royal Colleges of Physicians of London, Glasgow and Edinburgh. The particular requirements of paediatricians in training were recognized in 1993 by the introduction of a paediatric option for the MRCP part 1 multiple choice examination, to complement the part 2 examination in paediatrics. These are now being replaced in stages by parts 1 and 2 of the MRCPCH examination.

This book is arranged into five practice examinations, in the style of the paediatric option set by the Colleges. We have tried to establish a typical spread of subjects based on discussions with past candidates and on the specimen paper published by the Royal Colleges of Physicians in 1993. In particular, we have included representative proportions of questions relevant to general medicine and basic science questions, many of these applied to clinical situations. All of these questions are relevant to paediatrics.

As well as a self-assessment aid, this book is intended as a source of information. Each answer is accompanied by revision notes. More detail is provided for those answers which may be more difficult to find in standard texts. For candidates needing practice in specific areas we have included an index and have also compiled a separate contents by subject list. Some topics come under the umbrella of more than one subject heading and may therefore be listed several times.

All of our questions have been checked and rechecked against standard texts, and about half of them have been tried out on examination candidates. While we have eliminated questions that have been found to be wide open to individual interpretation, this exercise of checking and review has revealed the extreme difficulty of setting questions in medicine with unambiguous true/false answers. If the questions in this book are as good or better in this respect than those set by the examiners, then we will have achieved our aims.

We would like to acknowledge the assistance of those candidates who tried out our questions and gave us useful feedback in return, and of colleagues who provided helpful comments. There is no doubt that our families have benefited the least from this book and we would like to thank them above all for their patience throughout its preparation.

Jane Lucas
James Nicholson

Contents by subject

Anatomy
A1 A2 A60 B1 C1 C40 D1 E1 E4
Biochemistry and metabolic disease
A3 A4 A15 B2 B3 C2 C3 C17 C57 D2 D3 D15 E2 E3
Cardiology
A5 A6 A7 B4 B5 B6 B7 C4 C5 C6 C7 C46 C60 D2 D4 D5 D6
D7 D15 E4 E5 E6 E7 E57
Dermatology
A8 B8 B20 C8 D8
Development
A9 A10 B9 B10 C9 C10 D9 D10 E8 E9
Embryology
A11 B11 C11 D11 E10
Emergencies and poisoning
A5 A12 B12 C12 D12 E11 E47
Endocrinology
A13 A14 B2 B13 B14 B15 B16 C13 C14 C15 C16 D13 D14 D15
D16 D57 E12 E13 E14 E15
Gastroenterology and hepatology
A11 A16 A17 A18 A19 A36 B17 B18 B19 B34 C17 C18 C19 C20
D17 D18 D19 D20 D55 E16 E17 E18 E36
Genetics and inherited disorders
A10 A14 A20 A21 A22 A24 B20 B21 B22 B40 C2 C10 C17 C21
C22 C23 C33 C42 C53 D21 D22 D23 D44 E5 E18 E20 E21 E22 E43
Haematology
A23 A24 A25 A26 A32 B23 B24 B25 B45 C24 C25 C26 D24 D25
D26 E23 E24 E25 E49
Immunology
A23 A27 A28 A32 A59 B25 B26 B27 B28 C28 C29 C30 D27 D28
D29 D30 E26 E27 E28
Infectious diseases
A28 A29 A30 A31 A40 B5 B29 B30 B31 B32 B42 B54 B59 C5
C29 C30 C31 C32 C35 D30 D31 D32 D33 D51 E29 E30 E31 E32
Musculoskeletal system
B15 B33 C33 D33 E33 E55
Neonatology and fetal medicine
A6 A32 A34 A35 A36 B2 B27 B34 B35 B36 B37 B56 B59 C2 C6
C13 C19 C30 C34 C35 C36 C37 C43 C45 D24 D35 D36 D37 D45
E4 E7 E23 E35 E36 E37 E45
Nephrology
A37 A38 A39 B38 B39 C38 C39 C40 D38 D39 D47 E38 E39
Neurology
A1 A40 A41 A42 A60 B1 B40 B41 B42 B60 C1 C41 C42 C44 D1
D40 D41 D42 D58 E1 E10 E35 E40 E41 E44 E58

Nutrition
A43 B43 B44 C43 C55 D38 D43 E42
Oncology
A44 B25 B45 C44 D44 D48 D58 E26 E43
Ophthalmology
A45 B46 C45 C58 D59 E44
Pharmacology
A46 A47 A48 A49 B47 B48 B49 B50 C12 C32 C46 C47 C48 C49
D35 D45 D46 D47 D48 D49 D60 E45 E46 E47 E48 E49
Physiology
A7 A18 A54 A58 B3 B14 B16 B36 B39 B52 B53 B58 C7 C15 C16
C20 C40 C50 C54 C60 D7 D14 D15 D16 D18 D19 D53 E15 E17
E34 E40 E41 E53
Psychiatry
A15 A50 B51 C51 C59 D50 E50 E59
Respiratory
A35 A51 A52 A53 A54 A58 B37 B52 B53 B54 B58 C37 C48 C52
C53 C54 D3 D51 D52 D53 D60 E11 E18 E34 E37 E51 E52 E53
E54
Social paediatrics
A55 B55 C38 C55 D50 D54
Statistics and epidemiology
A33 A57 B56 B57 C56 D34 D56 E56
Surgery
A56 B18 B19 B34 C36 D36 D55 E36

Practice examination A   Questions

A1   Damage to the 2nd sacral nerve root may interfere with

A   hip flexion
B   the ankle jerk
C   sensation to the sole of the foot — S1 —
D   penile erection Parasymp +
E   relaxation of the detrusor muscle of the bladder —

A2   Concerning teeth

A   dentine is made principally of hydroxyapatite crystals
B   dentine has an abundant supply of blood vessels
C   no more enamel is made once the tooth has erupted
D   there are 28 deciduous teeth in a child 20- 32 Permant
E   the deciduous central incisors usually erupt at 6–8 months

A3   Hyperammonaemia may be caused by

A   severe burns
B   Reye's syndrome
C   ornithine transcarbamylase deficiency
D   liver disease
E   acute renal failure

A4   Blood gas analysis

A   of an infant with pyloric stenosis reveals a metabolic acidosis
B   of a child with diabetic ketoacidosis shows a base deficit
C   in salicylate poisoning may show a combination of respiratory alkalosis and metabolic acidosis
D   reveals an increased pH in acute respiratory failure
E   in partially compensated respiratory acidosis reveals a base deficit

A5   Electromechanical dissociation may result from

A   hypokalaemia
B   overdose with calcium channel blockers
C   tension pneumothorax
D   pericardial tamponade
E   hypoglycaemia

A6 Cyanosis is usual in the newborn period with

   A   Fallot's tetralogy
   B   transposition of the great arteries
   C   pulmonary atresia
   D   coarctation of the aorta
   E   endocardial fibroelastosis

A7 In recording of the central venous pressure

   A   the pressure is increased during inspiration
   B   the 'a' wave is caused by atrial systole
   C   the 'c' wave is caused by the bulging of the tricuspid valve during ventricular contraction
   D   the 'a' wave is prominent in pulmonary hypertension
   E   'a' waves are absent in complete heart block

A8 The following skin lesions are recognized associations of the conditions with which they are paired:

   A   dermatitis herpetiformis – coeliac disease
   B   shagreen patches – neurofibromatosis
   C   erythema multiforme – mycoplasma infection
   D   cavernous haemangioma – Kasabach–Merritt syndrome
   E   pyoderma gangrenosum – diabetes mellitus

A9 A normal 2 year old would be expected to

   A   walk downstairs, two feet per step
   B   identify three colours
   C   hold a simple conversation
   D   be mainly dry by day
   E   build a tower of six 2.5 cm cubes

A10 A 12 month old presents with a large head. Possible causes are

   A   large parental head size
   B   Down's syndrome
   C   achondroplasia
   D   Russell–Silver syndrome
   E   craniosynostosis

A11 During the development of the digestive system

   A the stomach develops from the foregut
   B mesodermal structures give rise to the peritoneum
   C the primitive intestinal loop normally rotates through 90° counterclockwise
   D the hindgut is temporarily connected to the yolk sac by means of the vitelline duct
   E anal atresia results from failure of division of the cloacal membrane

A12 The following would be appropriate for resuscitation of a 5 year old weighing 20 kg:

   A an endotracheal tube with an internal diameter of 7.0 mm
   B a 500 ml resuscitation bag
   C 2 ml of 1 in 10 000 adrenaline
   D initial defibrillation of 600 J
   E initial fluid infusion of 50 ml of colloid for a child with hypovolaemic shock

A13 The following may present with ambiguous genitalia:

   A Turner syndrome
   B congenital adrenal hyperplasia
   C panhypopituitarism
   D 5α-reductase deficiency
   E complete androgen insensitivity syndrome (CAIS)

A14 Causes of disproportionate short stature include

   A cystic fibrosis
   B septo-optic dysplasia
   C hypochondroplasia
   D untreated precocious puberty
   E hurler syndrome

A15 Laboratory investigations in anorexia nervosa may reveal

   A raised luteinizing hormone
   B exaggerated diurnal variation in cortisol levels
   C hypokalaemia
   D low somatomedin
   E hypoglycaemia

A16 Causes of diarrhoea include

- A   hypoparathyroidism
- B   Hirschsprung's disease
- C   hypothyroidism
- D   abetalipoproteinaemia
- E   total body irradiation prior to bone marrow transplantation

A17 The following are causes of prolonged neonatal conjugated hyperbilirubinaemia:

- A   congenital toxoplasmosis
- B   breast milk jaundice
- C   hypothyroidism
- D   cystic fibrosis
- E   Gilbert's syndrome

A18 Absorption of iron from the gastrointestinal tract is increased by

- A   iron deficiency
- B   antacids
- C   ascorbic acid
- D   growth hormone
- E   presence in ferrous form

A19 A thriving 10-year-old girl presents with recurrent abdominal pain.

- A   There is a 10% chance of an underlying organic cause
- B   An organic cause is likely if the pain is associated with vomiting
- C   Pallor associated with each painful episode is an indication for gastroscopy
- D   The differential diagnosis includes hereditary coproporphyria
- E   In the absence of vaginal bleeding, menstruation can be excluded as a cause

A20 The following are inherited in an autosomal dominant manner:

- A   galactosaemia
- B   Huntingdon's chorea
- C   benign essential tremor
- D   meningomyelocoele
- E   Fabry disease

A21 Features of Prader–Willi syndrome include

    A failure to thrive in infancy
    B hypotonia
    C large feet
    D hypogonadism
    E uniparental disomy

A22 In cytogenetic analysis

    A chromosome 3 is longer than chromosome 14
    B the nomenclature 11p refers to the long arm of chromosome 11
    C karyotyping of cells is facilitated by Giemsa staining of chromosomes
    D the Philadelphia chromosome may be denoted by t(9;22)
    E a deletion of the short arm of chromosome 5 is consistent with cri du chat syndrome

A23 A raised eosinophil count may be seen in

    A trichinosis
    B Hodgkin's disease
    C tuberculosis
    D corticosteroid therapy
    E polyarteritis nodosa

A24 In glucose-6-phosphate dehydrogenase (G6PD) deficiency

    A the pattern of inheritance is X-linked recessive
    B the direct Coombs' test is positive
    C cholesterol gallstones are a recognized complication
    D salicylates are safe
    E nitrofurantoin should be avoided

A25 Recognized causes of hyposplenism include

    A hereditary spherocytosis
    B chronic alcoholism
    C sickle cell disease
    D nephrotic syndrome
    E cystic fibrosis

A26 Causes of a prolonged bleeding time include

    A   haemolytic uraemic syndrome
    B   von Willebrand's disease
    C   classical haemophilia
  √ D   idiopathic thrombocytopenic purpura
  √ E   vitamin K deficiency

A27 IgA deficiency

    A   typically leads to severe sinopulmonary infections
    B   is associated with autoimmune disease
    C   should be treated with intravenous immunoglobulin therapy
    D   is a feature of hereditary angio-oedema
    E   is associated with atopy

A28 A live vaccine should not be given to a patient who

    A   is finishing a course of antibiotic treatment
    B   received pooled immunoglobulin 2 months ago
    C   has a previous history of the infection
    D   is receiving high-dose corticosteroids
    E   finished treatment for Hodgkin's disease 5 years ago

A29 *Staphylococcus aureus* is the most common causative organism in

    A   erythema toxicum
    B   Ritter's disease
    C   infected eczema
    D   acute osteomyelitis
    E   colonization of ventriculoperitoneal shunts

A30 Rubella

    A   has an incubation period of 7–10 days
    B   in children is usually preceded by a significant prodromal illness
    C   rarely results in a temperature more than 38°C in children
    D   may be complicated by a polyarthritis
    E   may be complicated by encephalitis

A31 Lyme disease

   A   is caused by *Borrelia burgdorferi*
   B   produces a characteristic rash of erythema marginatum
   C   typically affects the valves if the heart is involved
   D   can be diagnosed by enzyme linked immunosorbent assay (ELISA)
   E   should be treated with tetracycline in older children and adults

A32 Features of neonatal jaundice caused by ABO incompatibility include

   A   presentation in the first 24 h of life
   B   primiparous mother
   C   negative direct Coombs' test
   D   maternal blood group AB Rhesus negative
   E   direct bilirubin of 100 μmol/l (6 mg/100 ml)

A33 The following statements regarding mortality are true:

   A   an infant born at 23 weeks' gestation who lives for less than 1 h is classified as a stillbirth
   B   perinatal mortality rate includes stillbirths of more than 28 weeks' gestation
   C   a term infant who dies at 2 weeks of age is included in neonatal but not perinatal mortality figures
   D   an infant born at 34 weeks' gestation who dies at 5 weeks of age is classified as a neonatal death
   E   low birthweight infants (<2500 g) account for up to 20% of infant mortality in developed countries

A34 Alphafetoprotein is elevated in maternal serum when the fetus has

   A   gastroschisis
   B   Down's syndrome
   C   isolated hydrocephalus
   D   twin pregnancy
   E   congenital nephrotic syndrome

A35 In patients with bronchopulmonary dysplasia

A mechanical ventilation is an absolute prerequisite to developing the disease
B oxygen therapy is always indicated as part of the treatment
C hypercapnia should be avoided
D chest X-ray shows small lung fields with generalized opacification
E life expectancy is normal if the infant survives to leave hospital

A36 The following require investigation in an exclusively breast fed neonate:

A bright green stools
B blood in the stool on day 4 of life
C ten loose stools daily
D one loose stool every 4 days
E no meconium passed by 48 h

A37 Membranous nephropathy is associated with

A hepatitis B infection
B systemic lupus erythematosus
C HLA DR3
D diffuse proliferative changes on renal biopsy
E spontaneous remission

A38 In patients with haemolytic uraemic syndrome (HUS)

A thrombocytosis causes thrombotic occlusion of small blood vessels
B outlook is improved following early treatment with antibiotics
C an upper respiratory prodrome may precede the illness
D blood transfusions should be avoided
E prostacyclin activity is low

A39 Infantile polycystic renal disease

A is usually inherited as an X-linked recessive disease
B characteristically causes maternal polyhydramnios
C is associated with hepatic fibrosis
D has a high infant mortality
E can occur as unilateral disease

A40 Complications of bacterial meningitis include

A subdural haematoma
B hydrocephalus
C partial seizures
D sensorineural deafness
E diabetes insipidus

A41 Benign intracranial hypertension

A is a syndrome of asymptomatic raised intracranial pressure
B may follow head injury
C is a recognized complication of polycythaemia
D occurs more frequently in obese individuals
E may be associated with unilateral papilloedema

A42 Infantile spasms

A occur predominantly in the first year of life
B have a characteristic EEG showing hypsarrhythmia
C often have a strong family history
D may be treated with steroids
E have a good long-term outcome

A43 Kwashiorkor

A is often precipitated by weaning
B presents with oedema due to a protein losing enteropathy
C is associated with atrophy of the pancreas
D causes skin changes mainly on the arms and face
E results in body weight typically less than 60% of expected

A44 A thoracic mass, localized on lateral chest radiograph to the anterior mediastinum, is unlikely to be a

A non-Hodgkin's lymphoma
B neuroblastoma
C ganglioneuroma
D rhabdomyosarcoma
E cystic hygroma

A45 Cataracts occur in

- A Down's syndrome
- B cytomegalovirus infection
- C diabetes mellitus
- D congenital rubella syndrome
- E Lowe syndrome

A46 Infusion of 8.4% sodium bicarbonate solution may lead to

- A hypernatraemia
- B hypercalcaemia
- C intracellular acidosis
- D hypokalaemia
- E impaired tissue oxygen delivery

A47 Cisapride

- A is a weak dopamine receptor antagonist
- B increases resting tone in the lower oesophageal sphincter
- C may lead to constipation
- D is excreted unchanged by the kidneys
- E should not be given together with ketoconazole

A48 Paracetamol

- A shows cross sensitivity with 40% of patients who are allergic to aspirin
- B has no adverse effect on the liver unless taken in overdose
- C is converted to the toxic metabolite glutathione
- D overdose can be treated with an intravenous bolus of *N*-acetylcysteine
- E overdose should be monitored by liver enzyme assays

A49 H$_2$ antagonists

- A bind to receptors on gastric parietal cells
- B cross the blood–brain barrier
- C increase gastric emptying time
- D reduce pancreatic secretions
- E inhibit release of histamine

A50 Characteristic features of bulimia nervosa include

A preoccupation with food
B obesity
C amenorrhoea
D onset in early adolescence
E hypokalaemia

A51 A pleural effusion

A associated with pneumonic consolidation is likely to be caused by infection with *Mycoplasma pneumoniae*
B may be associated with mediastinal shift towards the affected side on plain chest radiograph
C may be chylous secondary to non-Hodgkin's lymphoma
D shows lymphocyte predominance and a low protein content in tuberculosis
E is very rarely found in children with connective tissue disorders

A52 The following statements are true of sweat tests:

A a sodium concentration of 70 mmol/l or more is indicative of cystic fibrosis (CF)
B they should be performed on newborn infants with meconium ileus to confirm the diagnosis of CF
C atropine is used topically to stimulate sweat production
D they are positive in more than 95% of children homozygous for CF
E the sweat test is useful in the identification of CF heterozygotes

A53 The following are commonly seen in asthma:

A wheeze during viral infections in an infant who is usually symptom-free
B monophonic wheeze on auscultation
C negative skin prick testing to common allergens in a 6 year old
D unilateral hyperlucency on chest X-ray
E segmental atelectasis on chest X-ray

A54 Changes associated with high altitude include

A   a decrease in the atmospheric concentration of oxygen
B   increased plasma volume
C   respiratory alkalosis
D   shift to the left of the oxyhaemoglobin dissociation curve
E   pulmonary vasoconstriction

A55 Radiographic changes strongly suggestive of non-accidental injury include

A   spiral fracture of the humerus
B   anterior rib fractures
C   linear fracture of the parietal bone
D   metaphyseal fracture of the knee
E   clavicular fracture

A56 A scrotal swelling

A   caused by an inguinal hernia is more likely to occur on the right than on the left
B   that transilluminates brightly in a 2-week-old infant should be explored surgically as soon as is practicable
C   associated with acute scrotal pain in a prepubertal boy is most likely to be caused by torsion of a testicular appendage
D   due to idiopathic scrotal oedema will be associated with testicular tenderness
E   resulting from epididymo-orchitis is most likely to be caused by infection with the mumps virus

A57 In the measurement of central tendency in a distribution of values

A   the mode does not exist if all values occur with the same frequency
B   the median is an unhelpful measure in a skewed distribution
C   of the mean, median and mode, the mean is the only measure which is amenable to mathematical operations
D   50% of observations fall above and below the median
E   the geometric mean is always smaller than the arithmetic mean

A58 Shunting of blood in the lungs

    A   describes the blood which enters the arterial system without passing through ventilated alveoli

    B   includes blood which passes through bronchial veins into pulmonary veins

    C   causes a raised carbon dioxide

    D   causes a hypoxia which cannot be abolished by 100% oxygen

    E   occurs in asthma

A59 With respect to complement,

    A   C2 is common to the classical and alternative pathways

    B   inherited deficiency of C5 is associated with meningococcal infection

    C   C3 levels are depressed in acute nephritis

    D   there is an increased incidence of sarcoidosis in people with complement deficiency

    E   deficiency is associated with autoimmune disease

A60 Stimulation of the parasympathetic nervous system leads to the following responses:

    A   increased salivary gland secretion

    B   gluconeogenesis

    C   miosis

    D   relaxation of the bladder sphincter

    E   gallbladder relaxation

Detrussor contracts

tongue relaxes,

contraction of Gb

Practice examination B   Questions

B1   A lesion of the ulnar nerve at the elbow may lead to

    A   inability to oppose the thumb and forefinger
    B   wrist drop
    C   unopposed flexion of the fourth and fifth metacarpophalangeal joints
    D   wasting of the muscles of the hypothenar eminence
    E   loss of sensation on the medial side of the dorsum and palm of the hand

B2   Causes of neonatal hypoglycaemia include

    A   erythroblastosis fetalis
    B   glycogen storage disease type 1
    C   maternal treatment with sodium valproate
    D   galactosaemia
    E   congenital adrenal hypoplasia

B3   In metabolic acidosis

    A   the blood pH is raised
    B   plasma bicarbonate is always reduced
    C   the base excess is negative
    D   plasma ionized calcium falls
    E   acetazolamide is a suitable treatment

B4   Hypertrophy of the cardiac septum

    A   in neonates may be caused by maternal diabetes mellitus
    B   rarely presents before middle age
    C   is associated with mitral regurgitation in the majority of cases
    D   may precede neurological manifestations of Friedreich's ataxia
    E   may be effectively treated with propranolol

B5   Infective endocarditis

    A   is most likely to occur before the age of 2 years in a patient at risk
    B   may occur in patients with a structurally normal heart
    C   is most commonly caused by β-haemolytic streptococci
    D   is associated with haematuria in one third of cases
    E   commonly leads to massive splenomegaly

B6   During a hypercyanotic attack in Fallot's tetralogy

A   a clinically pink child may become deeply cyanosed
B   there is increased right to left shunting of blood
C   the heart murmur may lessen in intensity
D   intravenous atropine may stop the episode
E   the infant should be placed in the recovery position

B7   The following are causes of pulmonary hypertension

A   pulmonary atresia
B   large tonsils
C   cystic fibrosis
D   coeliac disease
E   Fallot's tetralogy

B8   Causes of erythema multiforme include

A   infectious mononucleosis
B   orf
C   histoplasmosis
D   chlamydia infection
E   non-steroidal anti-inflammatory drugs

B9   The following reflexes are normally present at birth in a term neonate:

A   Moro
B   forward parachute
C   asymmetrical tonic neck reflex
D   glabellar tap
E   downgoing plantar

B10 At 36 months of age a normal child can

A   hop
B   kick a ball
C   give his name and sex
D   use a knife and fork competently
E   copy a circle

B11 The following structures are derived from endoderm:

A parathyroid glands
B spleen
C bladder
D pituitary gland
E inner ear

B12 Following the accidental ingestion of iron

A serum levels do not rise for the first 2 h
B circulatory failure may occur in the early stages
C metabolic alkalosis is a recognized complication
D desferrioxamine should be given intravenously in severe cases
E gastrointestinal obstruction may occur as a late effect

B13 Congenital adrenal hyperplasia

A is most commonly the result of 11 β-hydroxylase deficiency
B is more likely to present as a salt losing crisis in males than females
C shows autosomal recessive inheritance
D should be treated with fluid restriction in cases of hyponatraemia
E may be diagnosed and treated antenatally

B14 IGF-1 (insulin-like growth factor)

A is a glycoprotein
B acts as an antagonist to somatomedin C
C mediates growth promoting effects of human growth hormone
D is synthesized in largest quantities by the liver
E has no effect on blood sugar levels

B15 Causes of delayed bone age include

A familial short stature
B coeliac disease
C cranial irradiation
D hyperthyroidism
E Klinefelter syndrome

B16 The following hormones are released by the anterior lobe of pituitary

A calcitonin
B somatotrophin
C oxytocin
D prolactin
E antidiuretic hormone

B17 Raised serum conjugated bilirubin is associated with

A Rotor syndrome
B paroxysmal nocturnal haemoglobinuria
C hepatitis C infection
D haemochromatosis
E presence of bilirubin in the urine

B18 A 9-year-old girl presents with abdominal pain and blood in the stool. Possible causes include

A mesenteric adenitis
B necrotizing enterocolitis
C Meckel's diverticulitis
D Henoch-Schönlein purpura
E acute intermittent porphyria

B19 Intussusception

A has a peak incidence at 12–15 months
B is usually ileocolic
C usually has an underlying abnormality found at laparotomy
D occurs more commonly in patients with cystic fibrosis
E is the most common cause of intestinal obstruction under the age of 2 years

B20 Tuberous sclerosis is associated with

A adenomata of the sebaceous glands on the face
B renal cortical cysts
C cyanotic attacks in the newborn period
D polyostotic fibrous dysplasia
E deletions on the short arm of chromosome 16

B21 The following conditions are subject to X-linked recessive inheritance:

A   haemophilia B
B   nephrogenic diabetes insipidus
C   vitamin D dependent rickets
D   Hurler's syndrome
E   Holt Oram syndrome

B22 During normal somatic cell division

A   prophase marks the end of the resting phase (G_0) of the cell cycle
B   DNA replication is complete prior to the start of mitosis
C   sister chromatids are lined up during metaphase
D   treatment of cells with colchicine arrests dividing cells in anaphase
E   each nuclear envelope contains only one complete copy of genomic DNA at the end of telophase

B23 Causes of hypochromic red cells on the blood film include

A   coeliac disease
B   hiatus hernia
C   sickle cell disease
D   alpha thalassaemia trait
E   chronic inflammatory disease

B24 The following tests are normal in haemophilia A:

A   prothrombin time
B   fibrinogen
C   partial thromboplastin time
D   platelets
E   factor IX

B25 Blood products should be irradiated prior to transfusion in the following situations:

A   IgA deficiency
B   following bone marrow transplant
C   patients with DiGeorge syndrome
D   following induction chemotherapy for acute lymphoblastic leukaemia
E   patients with HIV infection

B26 Kawasaki disease

A leads to thrombocytopenia
B is diagnosed by viral titres
C is associated with desquamation of the palms
D is more common in girls
E should be treated with gammaglobulin infusions to reduce the incidence of coronary artery aneurysms

B27 A healthy term neonate differs from an adult in the following ways:

A less complement
B decreased IgG levels
C fewer B lymphocytes
D lower levels of secretory IgA
E a higher level of C reactive protein

B28 The following are causes of secondary immunodeficiency:

A nephrotic syndrome
B treatment with sodium valproate
C myotonic dystrophy
D sickle cell disease
E congenital rubella

B29 Toxoplasmosis may lead to

A asymptomatic infection
B chorioretinitis
C arthritis
D lymphopenia
E recurrence of the congenital infection in subsequent pregnancies

B30 The following are notifiable diseases in the UK

A whooping cough
B hepatitis A
C hand, foot and mouth disease
D HIV infection
E acute encephalitis

B31 The following incubation times are consistent with the infections with which they are paired

A   chicken pox – 21 days
B   whooping cough caused by *Bordetella pertussis* – 10 days
C   herpes simplex virus – 4 days
D   measles – 18 days
E   hand, foot and mouth disease – 14 days

B32 Adenovirus is a recognized cause of

A   bronchiolitis
B   gastroenteritis
C   myocarditis
D   haematuria
E   slapped cheek disease

B33 Systemic onset juvenile chronic arthritis is characterized by

A   presentation as a pyrexia of unknown origin
B   a vibratory midsystolic murmur at the lower left sternal edge
C   the presence of antinuclear antibody in the serum
D   iridocyclitis
E   a maculopapular rash

B34 Necrotizing enterocolitis (NEC) is a recognized complication of

A   polycythaemia
B   umbilical arterial catheterization
C   parenteral feeding
D   maternal Crohn's disease
E   birth asphyxia in a term neonate

B35 Hydrops fetalis may be associated with

A   Rhesus isoimmunization
B   paroxysmal supraventricular tachycardia
C   cytomegalovirus infection
D   achondroplasia
E   renal vein thrombosis

B36 Renal immaturity in normal neonates born at term is manifest as

A   a reduced number of nephrons
B   decreased glucose reabsorption
C   increased glomerular filtration rate
D   decreased renal bicarbonate reabsorption
E   decreased urea excretion

B37 The following maternal factors increase the incidence of surfactant deficient respiratory distress syndrome:

A   steroid therapy
B   opiates
C   placental insufficiency, leading to intrauterine growth retardation
D   diabetes
E   alcoholism

B38 In minimal change nephrotic syndrome

A   there may be intravascular volume depletion
B   increased secretion of antidiuretic hormone may occur
C   the course of the disease should be monitored by frequent serum albumin estimations
D   concentrated albumin infusions are required in the majority of cases
E   70% achieve permanent remission with oral corticosteroids

B39 Glomerular filtration rate

A   should be measured using a substance which is reabsorbed by the tubules
B   requires collection of both blood and urine for measurement
C   is reduced by efferent arteriolar constriction
D   is reduced by sympathetic nervous stimulation
E   may be reduced by treatment with cisplatin

B40 Rett syndrome

A   affects males and females in equal numbers
B   is inherited in an autosomal dominant manner
C   presents with developmental delay in the first 6 months of life
D   leads to the loss of purposeful hand movements
E   is associated with microcephaly

B41 Primary generalized absence seizures

A   are characterized by an electroencephalograph showing spike and wave activity at 3 cycles/s
B   are typically not preceded by an aura
C   usually last 2–3 minutes
D   should be treated with phenobarbitone
E   are rarely associated with the development of generalized tonic-clonic seizures

B42 Subacute sclerosing panencephalitis

A   usually occurs 5–10 years following infection with measles
B   is associated with high levels of measles antibody in the serum
C   is typically associated with three per second spike and wave activity on the electroencephalogram
D   is characterized by preservation of intellectual ability until the late stages of disease
E   has had a lower incidence in the population since the introduction of measles vaccination

B43 Thiamine (vitamin B₁) deficiency

A   is slow to develop because of the size of body stores
B   is rare if the staple diet contains legumes and pulses
C   results in inadequate metabolism of glucose
D   results in pellagra
E   with severe oedema, typically responds to appropriate treatment within hours

B44 The following are true of breast milk:

A   maternal malnutrition has a negligible effect on the protein content of milk
B   it contains less calcium than cow's milk
C   it may protect against haemorrhagic disease of the newborn
D   specific passive immunity is conferred by IgA
E   breast feeding favours gut colonization by *Escherichia coli*

B45 The following are indicators of a relatively poor prognosis at the diagnosis of acute lymphoblastic leukaemia:

A   leucocyte count less than $4 \times 10^9/l$
B   male sex
C   age above 2 years
D   thrombocytopenia
E   T cell markers on the blast cells

B46 Amblyopia

A   may be caused by congenital cataract
B   may be associated with abnormal head posture
C   is a frequent complication of paralytic squint
D   is diagnosed using the cover test
E   usually resolves spontaneously in preschool children

B47 The following antimicrobials are bactericidal:

A   benzyl penicillin
B   cephaclor
C   tobramycin
D   trimethoprim
E   doxycycline

B48 Alprostadil (prostaglandin E₁)

A   is used in neonates to close a patent ductus arteriosus
B   is administered by slow intravenous bolus
C   causes apnoea
D   inhibits the action of dopamine
E   may lead to gastric outflow obstruction

B49 When prescribing

A   0.1 mg (milligrams) is equivalent to 100 µg (micrograms)
B   0.02 µg is equivalent to 200 ng (nanograms)
C   1 ml (millilitre) of adrenaline 1:1000 contains 0.1 mg of adrenaline
D   sodium bicarbonate 8.4% contains 1 mmol/ml
E   glucose 4% with saline 0.18% contains approximately 150 mmol/l of sodium

B50 Morphine

    A increases the secretion of antidiuretic hormone
    B leads to contraction of the sphincter of Oddi
    C causes coughing
    D decreases gastric acid secretion
    E leads to histamine release

B51 Features of anorexia nervosa include

    A increased incidence in lower social classes
    B delusions of fatness
    C alopecia
    D avoidance of fluids
    E sensitivity to cold

B52 The oxyhaemoglobin dissociation curve is shifted to the right by

    A a decrease in temperature
    B an increase in 2,3 diphosphoglycerate in the erythrocytes
    C fetal haemoglobin
    D hypercarbia
    E haemoglobin S

B53 Hyperventilation in the ventilated patient

    A lowers the pH of blood
    B is a cause of tetany
    C may be partially compensated by renal secretion of hydrogen ions
    D increases cerebral blood flow
    E reduces the plasma bicarbonate

B54 In patients with pneumonia

    A *Pneumococcus* is the bacterium most frequently identified in a previously well child
    B cytomegalovirus is a rare cause in otherwise healthy children
    C *Mycoplasma pneumoniae* typically causes more dramatic physical signs than the symptoms would suggest
    D *Staphylococcus* is a common cause in preschool children
    E *Pneumocystis carinii* responds to treatment with co-trimoxazole

B55 Following the Children Act (1989)

A   parental responsibility is automatically shared by both parents

B   an Emergency Protection Order may be enforced only by application to a magistrate's court

C   the maximum duration of Police Protection Provisions is 72 h

D   parental responsibility is transferred to the local authority during a Child Assessment Order

E   the wishes of the child may be decisive in care proceedings

B56 The following statements concerning screening tests are correct:

A   specificity of 90% implies a 10% false negative rate

B   a test with a predictive value of 85% will have a false positive rate of 15%

C   in the evaluation of a potential screening test, it is more important to minimize false positives than false negatives

D   the Guthrie test should be performed in newborn infants before milk feeds are fully established

E   cystic fibrosis can be diagnosed in the newborn period by screening infants for immunoreactive trypsin in the blood

B57 Where the correlation coefficient (*r*) is measured between variables *x* and *y*

A   the sampling distribution of *r* is normal

B   if $r = 1$, all values lie on a straight line

C   the larger the value of *r*, the greater the likelihood of a causative link between *x* and *y*

D   when $r = -1$, there is no correlation between *x* and *y*

E   the value of *r* equates to the gradient of the regression line for *x* and *y*

B58 Carbon dioxide

A   in the blood is transported mostly in solution

B   is displaced from haemoglobin in the lungs due to the Haldane effect

C   reacts with hydrogen ions in erythrocytes under the catalytic effect of carbonic anhydrase

D   is twenty times more soluble than oxygen

E   obeys Henry's law in the dissolved state

B59 Bacteria commonly isolated in cases of neonatal meningitis include

A   *Escherichia coli*
B   *Haemophilus influenzae*
C   Group B streptococcus
D   *Staphylococcus epidermidis*
E   *Neisseria meningitidis*

B60 Stimulation of β_2 receptors causes

A   relaxation of the gastrointestinal wall
B   uterine contraction
C   glycogenolysis
D   contraction of the detrusor muscle of the bladder
E   dilatation of arterioles in skeletal muscle

Practice examination C   Questions

C1 Unilateral transection of the spinal cord is likely to lead to

A upper motor neuron lesions of affected muscle groups

B weakness of voluntary movements of ipsilateral muscle groups supplied from below the level of the lesion

C impairment of temperature sensation on the same side as the lesion

D impaired perception of fine touch below and contralateral to the lesion

E suppression of the cremasteric reflex on the affected side if the lesion is above L1

C2 Galactosaemia

A is caused by deficiency of the enzyme galactokinase

B causes jaundice in the newborn

C may present with cataracts at birth

D is associated with *Escherichia coli* septicaemia

E is diagnosed as a result of screening in the majority of cases

C3 Vitamin D

A levels in breast milk are higher than in standard infant formulae

B circulates mainly in the form 1,25-dihydroxycholecalciferol

C in the form 24,25-dihydroxycholecalciferol, does not have an active role in calcium metabolism

D in its active form inhibits the action of parathyroid hormone on bone

E deficiency results in low plasma calcium levels and raised phosphate

C4 A murmur with the following features is unlikely to be innocent:

A presence in the aortic area

B radiation to the back

C presence of a thrill

D accentuation by fever

E vibratory quality

C5   Infective myocarditis

A   is most commonly due to infection with adenovirus
B   is a potential complication of bacteraemia
C   due to diphtheria toxin most commonly affects the conducting tissue of the heart
D   may result in chronic dilated cardiomyopathy
E   produces characteristic ECG changes

C6   Supraventricular tachycardia in neonates

A   is the most common abnormal tachycardia
B   reflects underlying congenital heart disease in the majority of cases
C   shows a regular rate of 160–220 beats per minute on the electrocardiogram
D   recurrent episodes usually persist into adulthood
E   may be stopped with a rapid intravenous bolus of adenosine

C7   The following are cardiac catheterization data from a 9-month-old boy. The oxygen saturation (%) is presented first, followed by the pressure (mmHg):

Right atrium 73% saturated, mean pressure 5 mmHg. Right ventricle 86%, 80/5 mmHg. Pulmonary artery 86%, 80/55 mmHg. Femoral artery 96%, 80/55 mmHg.

A   The child has a ventricular septal defect
B   There is significant pulmonary stenosis
C   The boy is likely to be centrally cyanosed
D   Corrective surgery is indicated
E   The arterial $P\text{CO}_2$ is likely to be significantly raised

C8   The following rashes usually resolve without treatment:

A   erythema multiforme
B   urticaria pigmentosa
C   eosinophilic granuloma
D   Henoch–Schönlein purpura
E   eczema herpeticum

C9   An average 12 month old will

A   walk with one hand held
B   have a vocabulary of six words
C   look for an object when it is moved out of sight
D   pick up 'hundreds and thousands' with a fine pincer grasp
E   wave

C10 The following conditions are associated with learning difficulties:

A   Turner syndrome
B   tuberous sclerosis
C   osteogenesis imperfecta tarda
D   Klinefelter syndrome
E   mucopolysaccharidosis type IV (Morquio disease)

C11 The mesodermal germ layer gives rise to

A   striated muscle
B   the spleen
C   the adrenal medulla
D   bone
E   the gastrointestinal tract

C12 Effects of acute theophylline poisoning include

A   vomiting
B   convulsions
C   hyperkalaemia
D   pupillary dilatation
E   ventricular arrhythmias

C13 Clinical features of congenital hypothyroidism diagnosed in the newborn period include

A   large tongue
B   presence of a third fontanelle
C   umbilical hernia
D   loose stools
E   a high incidence of mental retardation

C14 The onset of puberty

A   depends on the pulsatile secretion of gonadotrophin releasing hormone
B   in a boy before the age of 9 years should be investigated
C   is indicated by isolated breast development in a 2-year-old girl
D   is suggested by a testicular volume of 5 ml
E   is marked by a growth spurt in both sexes

C15 Growth hormone secretion is stimulated by

A   stress
B   pregnancy
C   hyperglycaemia
D   fasting
E   cortisol

C16 Insulin

A   promotes the use of fats for energy
B   controls glucose permeability of brain cell membranes
C   secretion is stimulated by acetylcholine
D   secretion is inhibited by α-agonists
E   is excreted unchanged by the kidneys

C17 Features consistent with the diagnosis of Wilson's disease include

A   Kayser–Fleischer rings
B   low urinary copper
C   normal serum copper
D   haemolysis
E   aminoaciduria

C18 A 3-year-old boy presents with failure to thrive and diarrhoea. Possible causes include

A   Crohn's disease
B   toddler diarrhoea
C   cystic fibrosis
D   Schwachmann's syndrome
E   idiopathic hypercalcaemia

C19 Causes of a persisting neonatal unconjugated hyperbilirubinaemia after 2 weeks include

A   rhesus incompatibility
B   hypothyroidism
C   breast milk jaundice
D   Rotor syndrome
E   sepsis

C20 Pancreatic juice contains

A trypsin
B cholecystokinin
C cholesterol esterase
D hydrochloric acid
E amylase

C21 Autosomal recessive conditions include

A Dubin–Johnson syndrome
B ataxia telangiectasia
C Wiskott–Aldrich syndrome
D hereditary spherocytosis
E Treacher–Collins syndrome

C22 Genetic anticipation is a feature of

A Huntington's disease
B fragile X syndrome
C Angelman syndrome
D Leber's optic atrophy
E myotonic dystrophy

C23 Features of Klinefelter syndrome include

A the karyotype 47XYY
B higher incidence of malignancy than in unaffected males
C short stature
D normal intellect
E large genitalia

C24 The following statements regarding haemoglobin and its subgroups are true:

A HbA is present throughout fetal life
B HbF declines to adult levels by 3 months of age
C HbA_2 is only present in patients with beta-thalassaemia
D Hb Barts is incompatible with extrauterine life
E haemoglobin electrophoresis of cord blood can be used to diagnose beta-thalassaemia

C25 Situations in which the prothrombin time is increased include

A use of oral anticoagulants
B von Willebrand's disease
C haemorrhagic disease of the newborn
D disseminated intravascular coagulation
E Christmas disease

C26 A reticulocyte count of more than 10% may be caused by

A Fanconi's anaemia
B thalassaemia intermedia
C hereditary spherocytosis
D glucose-6-phosphate dehydrogenase deficiency
E iron deficiency anaemia

C27 Henoch–Schönlein purpura

A is most common among preschool children
B typically produces a rash involving the lower limbs and buttocks
C is complicated by renal involvement in 5% of children
D may be complicated by intussusception
E is associated with thrombocytopenia

C28 Immunoglobulin G

A has a molecular weight of 900 000 dalton
B is the first immunoglobulin class to rise in acute infection
C has a half life of 21 days
D falls in the first few weeks of life
E is the main immunoglobulin class involved in the ABO blood group system

C29 The following are live attenuated vaccines:

A tetanus
B BCG
C typhoid
D *Haemophilus influenzae* B (Hib)
E measles

C30 Vertical transmission of the human immunodeficiency virus (HIV)

A   occurs only in the second and third trimesters
B   takes place in over 90% of affected pregnancies
C   is the most common route of infection in children
D   may be reduced by avoidance of breast feeding
E   can be excluded by a negative antibody test at 12 months of age

C31 Measles

A   is infectious 3 days before the onset of the rash
B   complicated by convulsions is suggestive of encephalitis
C   is associated with selective suboccipital lymphadenopathy
D   is always associated with conjunctivitis
E   is characterized by Koplik spots

C32 Advice regarding malaria prophylaxis should include the following:

A   chloroquine prophylaxis should not be used continuously for more than 1 year
B   corneal opacities due to prolonged chloroquine use disappear completely when the drug is stopped
C   chloroquine is excreted in breast milk making separate chemoprophylaxis unnecessary for the infant
D   prophylaxis should start 4 weeks before exposure to risk
E   prophylaxis should continue until 4 weeks after leaving the malarial region

C33 The following are causes of inequality of leg length:

A   tuberculosis
B   Klippel–Trenaunay syndrome
C   William's syndrome
D   Russell Silver syndrome
E   neurofibromatosis

C34 Growth retarded babies are at increased risk of

A   polycythaemia
B   hyaline membrane disease
C   hypoglycaemia
D   Group B streptococcal infection
E   sudden intrapartum death

C35 Congenital rubella

A is associated with cerebral calcification
B frequently leads to cataracts
C is associated with ventricular septal defects
D rarely occurs following maternal infection in the third trimester
E should be prevented by vaccinating women found to be seronegative during the first trimester

C36 Oesophageal atresia is associated with

A maternal hydramnios
B vertebral anomalies
C diaphragmatic hernia
D low birthweight
E duplex collecting system

C37 The following are causes of tachypnoea presenting in the first 72 h of life:

A Wilson–Mikity syndrome
B infantile polycystic renal disease
C bronchopulmonary dysplasia
D coarctation of the aorta
E aneurysm of the vein of Galen

C38 Nocturnal enuresis

A occurs with a frequency of 1% in 8 year olds
B is associated with a positive family history in 70% of cases
C may be the presenting feature of diabetes mellitus
D is an expected complication of a duplex collecting system
E is more common in girls than boys

C39 Haemolytic uraemic syndrome (HUS)

A occurs in summer epidemics
B usually follows infection with a verotoxin producing strain of *Shigella*
C gives a microangiopathic haemolytic picture on blood film
D is associated with neutrophilia
E is the commonest cause of acute renal failure in childhood

C40 The following are true of renal circulation:

A the renal medulla receives a much larger volume of blood per unit mass than the cortex

B para-aminohippuric acid may be used to measure renal blood flow in the older child

C the peritubular capillaries are at relatively high pressure

D hypoxia causes renal vasodilatation

E renal blood flow represents 20–25% of resting cardiac output

C41 Features of complex partial seizures include

A association with febrile illness

B auditory hallucinations

C vomiting

D no alteration in consciousness

E abnormal interictal EEG in the majority of cases

C42 Patients with Friedreich's ataxia

A may present with angina

B have an increased incidence of diabetes mellitus

C commonly have telangiectasia of the conjunctiva

D have brisk ankle reflexes

E often have dysarthria

C43 Human breast milk contains

A secretory IgA

B macrophages

C lysozyme

D vitamin C

E zinc

C44 In neuroblastoma

A there is a recognized association with Hirschsprung's disease

B the presence of raised urinary catecholamine metabolites is a prerequisite to diagnosis

C reduced plasma ferritin levels are found

D the prognosis is worse in infants under the age of 12 months

E spontaneous resolution may occur

C45 Retinopathy of prematurity

    A   develops in the first week of life
    B   is more likely to occur in very low birth weight infants
    C   is a recognized complication of hypoglycaemia
    D   rarely resolves spontaneously
    E   may be treated effectively with laser therapy

C46 In the treatment of hypertension

    A   captopril is particularly suited to use in patients with renal artery stenosis
    B   hydralazine may lead to the development of a lupus-like syndrome
    C   nifedipine is poorly absorbed enterally
    D   propranolol may exacerbate symptoms of asthma
    E   the use of phentolamine is limited to cases of catecholamine excess

C47 The first named of the following pairs of drugs may result in reduced plasma levels of the second:

    A   carbamezapine – warfarin
    B   cimetidine – propranolol
    C   phenobarbitone – aminophylline
    D   probenecid – penicillin
    E   aspirin – methotrexate

C48 Salbutamol

    A   is a selective β_1-agonist
    B   increases intracellular cyclic AMP levels
    C   given intravenously has little therapeutic benefit in the treatment of asthma
    D   acts only on the lung when administered by inhalation
    E   increases plasma potassium levels

C49 Ototoxicity from aminoglycosides may be exacerbated by

    A   birth asphyxia
    B   amphotericin B therapy
    C   frusemide therapy
    D   hypokalaemia
    E   mannitol

C50 A child with a body weight of 20 kg will have

A a total body water volume of 12–13 l
B a circulating blood volume of 2.5 l
C a daily urine output of 150–300 ml
D a daily maintenance fluid requirement of 1500 ml
E daily insensible fluid losses of 400–500 ml

C51 The following are associated with childhood autism:

A poor eye contact
B epilepsy
C social deprivation
D prevalence bias towards girls
E obsessional rituals

C52 Causes of acute onset of stridor include

A laryngomalacia
B foreign body inhalation
C infection with parainfluenza virus type III
D whooping cough
E hypoparathyroidism

C53 Cystic fibrosis (CF)

A results from a defect in the CF transmembrane regulator gene located on chromosome 7
B in a 2 year old is most reliably confirmed by direct gene analysis
C is rare in non-caucasians
D has an incidence of approximately 1 in 25 000 births in the UK
E is most commonly associated with a δ F 508 mutation

C54 In the assessment of lung function

A the vital capacity equals the inspiratory reserve volume plus the tidal volume plus the functional residual capacity
B the residual volume is the lung volume at the end of a normal breath
C the total lung capacity consists of the vital capacity plus the residual volume
D the functional residual capacity cannot be measured with a simple spirometer
E a flow volume curve can be plotted using a spirometer

C55 Causes of obesity in childhood include

A Prader–Willi syndrome
B clonazepam
C sodium valproate
D pseudohypoparathyroidism
E Laurence–Moon–Biedl syndrome

C56 In statistical analysis:

A a type I error is a hypothesis which is rejected when it is true
B standard deviation is a measure of the differences of each observation from the mean
C the standard deviation is the square of the variance
D the standard error of the mean is larger than the population standard deviation
E the probability of an impossible event occurring is $P = -1$

C57 Inappropriate antidiuretic hormone secretion

A results in hypotonic urine
B can be caused by the use of frusemide
C is a common complication of surgery requiring a general anaesthetic
D is often complicated by severe oedema
E can be treated by water restriction

C58 The following conditions increase the risk of a visual defect:

A conjunctival haemorrhages at birth
B pauciarticular onset juvenile chronic arthritis
C Apert's syndrome
D Henoch–Schönlein purpura
E galactosaemia

C59 Features of childhood complaints suggesting the non-organic origin of symptoms include

A headaches which occur daily and do not wake the child at night
B abdominal pain localized to one flank
C backache in a 5 year old
D restricted internal rotation about a painful hip joint
E generalized seizures which start abruptly

C60 The normal cardiac action potential

    A has a resting muscle transmembrane potential of -90 mV

    B exhibits spontaneous depolarization of contractile cells in phase 4

    C involves rapid movement of sodium into the cells during phase 0

    D has a change in transmembrane potential during phase 0 to a peak of $+90$ mV

    E has an absolute refractory period extending through phases 1, 2 and part of phase 3

Practice examination D   Questions

D1   Damage to the posterior interosseous nerve leads to

A   paralysis of extensor carpi radialis longus
B   paralysis of abductor pollicis longus
C   loss of the ability to pronate the forearm
D   anaesthesia over the lateral part of the dorsum of the hand
E   reduced nerve supply to the intercarpal joints

D2   Hypokalaemia and hypertension are recognized associations in

A   Addison's disease
B   21α-hydroxylase deficiency
C   adrenal adenoma
D   Bartter's syndrome
E   renal artery stenosis

D3   The following conditions are associated with raised sweat electrolytes:

A   hyperthyroidism
B   nephrogenic diabetes insipidus
C   adrenal insufficiency
D   infantile polycystic kidney disease
E   anorexia nervosa

D4   In the diagnosis and assessment of heart failure in infancy

A   profuse sweating may be the presenting symptom
B   the infant is frequently noted to feed hungrily
C   the neck should be observed carefully for jugular venous pressure
D   a heart rate greater than 180 beats per minute is suggestive of supraventricular tachycardia
E   the degree of hepatomegaly is related to the severity of the heart failure

D5   Prophylactic antibiotic cover should be given for dental procedures to individuals with the following cardiac lesions:

A   coarctation of the aorta
B   ligated patent ductus arteriosus
C   bicuspid aortic valve disease
D   hypertrophic cardiomyopathy
E   secundum atrial septal defect

D6 **The following are major criteria (revised Jones criteria 1984) for the diagnosis of rheumatic fever:**

A   prolonged PR interval
B   subcutaneous nodules
C   increased titre of anti-streptococcal antibodies
D   erythema nodosum
E   arthralgia

D7 **The second heart sound**

A   corresponds to closure of the aortic and pulmonary valves
B   coincides with the R wave on an electrocardiogram
C   is widely split in Fallot's tetralogy
D   is loud in a ventricular septal defect complicated by pulmonary hypertension
E   is split by a fixed interval in atrial septal defect

D8 **Features of skin conditions occurring in the newborn period include**

A   sparing of the skin creases in napkin candidiasis
B   an association between harlequin colour change and anomalous pulmonary venous drainage
C   resolution of naevus flammeus (port wine stain) in the first year of life
D   blistering from birth in epidermolysis bullosa
E   the appearance of erythema toxicum neonatorum at any time in the first 14 days of life

D9 **The following would be cause for concern in a 6-month-old infant:**

A   failure to crawl
B   persistence of the stepping reflex
C   no pincer grasp
D   failure to respond to mother's voice
E   mouthing of objects

D10 **The following are causes of speech delay:**

A   hypothyroidism *Retardation*
B   twins
C   subacute sclerosing panencephalitis *Regression*
D   tongue tie
E   phenylketonuria

D11 The following statements are true of normal sexual differentiation:

A the basic programmed pattern of development is female which is only overridden by the presence of a Y chromosome

B all embryos have both ovarian and testicular tissue prior to differentiation

C the majority of the process is complete by the end of the first trimester of pregnancy

D Müllerian inhibiting factor is secreted by the ovaries

E the conversion of testosterone to dihydrotestosterone is required for the normal development of external genitalia in a male

D12 Lead poisoning

A interferes with haem synthesis

B is associated with a low free erythrocyte protoporphyrin

C is associated with a high urinary delta aminolaevulinic acid

D can present with nephrogenic diabetes insipidus

E is usually complicated by diarrhoea

D13 In the assessment of stature

A a single measurement below the third centile warrants investigation

B growth velocity on the 25th centile will maintain height on the 25th centile

C projected height is calculated by taking the midpoint between parental heights

D bone age estimations are made from plain radiographs of the left wrist

E a normal growth hormone response to an exercise stress test excludes growth hormone deficiency

D14 The adrenal gland

A has no physiological role in the fetus

B secretes androgens from the zona glomerulosa

C produces cortisol in a pulsatile fashion, with morning dips in blood levels

D contributes little to the pool of circulating androgens in adolescent males

E is essential for the development of female pubic hair

D15 Atrial natriuretic factor

  A   is released in response to increased right atrial pressure
  B   is a vasodilator
  C   reduces urinary secretion of sodium
  D   antagonizes release of aldosterone
  E   is an inotrope

D16 Thyroid stimulating hormone

  A   is released from the hypothalamus
  B   secretion is inhibited by somatostatin
  C   activates cyclic adenosine monophosphate
  D   increases the uptake of iodide into the thyroid gland
  E   increases proteolysis of thyroglobulin in the thyroid
      follicles

D17 Extraintestinal manifestations of Crohn's disease include

  A   pubertal delay
  B   ankylosing spondylitis
  C   cataract
  D   chronic active hepatitis
  E   erythema multiforme

D18 The following statements about bilirubin formation and excretion are true:

  A   biliverdin is formed from haem
  B   most bilirubin circulates in the blood in an unbound
      form
  C   glucuronyl transferase is inhibited by steroids
  D   urobilinogen in the gut is reabsorbed
  E   in Gilbert's syndrome there is a defect in transportation
      of the conjugated bilirubin from the hepatocytes into the
      bile

D19 Gastric hydrogen ion secretion is

  A   the function of chief cells
  B   stimulated by histamine acting on histamine-2 receptors
  C   increased by secretin
  D   abolished by vagotomy
  E   necessary for protein digestion in the stomach

D20 Chronic duodenal ulcers in children

A   occur more frequently than chronic gastric ulcers
B   are often associated with a positive family history
C   are the most common cause of recurrent abdominal pain
D   may be caused by gastrin secreting tumours
E   should be diagnosed by endoscopy

D21 Down's syndrome

A   results more commonly from non-disjunction than translocation
B   accounts for 30% of cases of anal atresia
C   is frequently associated with significant hearing problems
D   predisposes individuals to Alzheimer's disease
E   in a fetus leads to lower than normal levels of unconjugated oestriol in maternal serum

D22 X-linked dominant conditions include

A   Becker muscular dystrophy
B   Tay–Sachs disease
C   familial hypercholesterolaemia
D   vitamin D-resistant rickets
E   ornithine transcarbamylase deficiency

D23 In an autosomal recessive condition

A   50% of the children of an affected mother will be affected
B   if both parents are carriers, all of the offspring will also be carriers
C   with a carrier rate of 1 in 50, the prevalence of the condition will be approximately 1 in 10 000
D   the affected individuals in a family are likely to be in one sibship
E   the incidence is increased in the offspring of consanguineous unions

D24 Causes of neonatal polycythaemia include

A   congenital rubella infection
B   pre-eclampsia
C   maternal diabetes mellitus
D   delayed clamping of the umbilical cord
E   congenital adrenal hyperplasia

D25 Von Willebrand disease

A   is inherited in an autosomal recessive manner
B   results from a functional abnormality in factor IX
C   may present with mucosal bleeding in the newborn
period
D   may be diagnosed antenatally by DNA analysis
E   in its most severe form, may be effectively treated using
DDAVP

D26 Splenomegaly and a normal white cell count are associated with

A   Fanconi's anaemia
B   lymphoma
C   hereditary spherocytosis
D   Hurler syndrome
E   sickle cell disease

D27 C reactive protein (CRP)

A   is synthesized in the liver
B   production is stimulated by interleukin-6
C   freely crosses the placenta
D   concentration rises following intraventricular haemor-
rhage in premature neonates
E   usually takes more than a week to return to normal
levels following clinical resolution of bacterial infection
in the newborn

D28 Interferon gamma

A   is produced mainly by fibroblasts
B   activates macrophages to kill intracellular bacteria
C   has an antiviral effect
D   shares a common receptor with interferon alpha
(INF-α)
E   is licensed for the treatment of hairy cell leukaemia

D29 Complement deficiency occurs in

A   systemic lupus erythematosus
B   hereditary angio-oedema
C   acute pancreatitis
D   membranoproliferative glomerulonephritis
E   sarcoidosis

D30 In children with HIV infection

A   thrombocytopenia may be the presenting feature
B   polyclonal hypergammaglobulinaemia is a recognized finding
C   Kaposi's sarcoma is relatively more common than in infected adults
D   routine immunizations should be withheld
E   the presence of p24 antibody is a poor prognostic indicator

D31 Features of typhoid fever include

A   infection with *Salmonella typhimurium*
B   an incubation period of 10–14 days
C   cough
D   a macular rash over the trunk
E   response to treatment with trimethoprim

D32 Mumps

A   is infectious from the first day of salivary gland swelling
B   leads to raised serum amylase
C   is rarely complicated by orchitis before puberty
D   may present with lymphocytic meningitis
E   can be effectively prevented using a killed vaccine

D33 An 18-month-old child presents with a 2-day history of fever and reluctance to bear weight on his right leg. Examination reveals exquisite tenderness over his right tibial metaphysis.

A   The most likely diagnosis is septic arthritis of the knee
B   Plain radiography has no place in the first week following presentation
C   The most likely causative organism is *Haemophilus influenzae* B
D   Treatment should be delayed until after microbiological confirmation of the diagnosis
E   With appropriate treatment, complete resolution without long-term complications is likely

D34 A district in which there are 4000 deliveries per annum could reasonably expect the following each year

A two new cases of cystic fibrosis
B two infants born with hypospadias
C a perinatal mortality rate of 7 per 1000
D two cases of haemorrhagic disease of the newborn
E fifty sets of twins conceived naturally

D35 Neonates suffering withdrawal from *in utero* exposure to narcotics may show signs of

A irritability
B vomiting
C photophobia
D hypotonia
E diarrhoea

D36 The following conditions may present with bile-stained vomiting in the first week of life:

A duodenal atresia
B cystic fibrosis
C inguinal hernia
D gastro-oesophageal reflux
E necrotizing enterocolitis

D37 Polyhydramnios is associated with

A oesophageal atresia
B Potter's syndrome
C anencephaly
D diaphragmatic hernia
E maternal diabetes

D38 In the dietary management of patients with renal disease, the following are appropriate:

A a high energy intake in acute renal failure
B high phosphate intake in chronic renal failure
C normal potassium intake in chronic renal failure
D increased salt in nephrotic syndrome
E normal protein intake in nephrotic syndrome

D39 Postinfectious glomerulonephritis

A   typically occurs following infection with Lancefield Group A β-haemolytic streptococcus
B   is most common in school age children
C   should be investigated with a renal biopsy when the diagnosis is suspected
D   may lead to blunting of the costophrenic angles on plain chest radiograph
E   should be treated with prednisolone

D40 Unilateral lower motor neuron facial nerve palsy

A   is a well-recognized presenting feature of hypertension
B   spares the upper part of the face
C   may be caused by a cerebral hemisphere tumour
D   persisting 3 weeks after birth trauma, is likely to be permanent
E   of undetermined cause may be successfully treated with corticosteroids

D41 The cerebrospinal fluid

A   is secreted from the arachnoid villi
B   has a normal pressure of 20 cm CSF in a recumbent 15 year old
C   is normally a pale yellow colour
D   contains a predominance of mononuclear white cells in tubercular meningitis
E   has a raised protein level in Guillain Barré syndrome

D42 Febrile convulsions

A   characteristically first occur under the age of 6 months
B   are associated with an increased risk of epilepsy
C   may be unilateral
D   are commonly followed by further convulsions in the same febrile illness
E   may occur with teething

D43 The following statements about vitamins are true:

A   vitamin A is destroyed by cooking
B   a deficiency of riboflavin causes glossitis and cheilosis
C   vitamin D is synthesized in the skin as 1, 25-dihydroxy-cholecalciferol
D   ileal resection leads to a deficiency of vitamin K
E   renal disease can result in vitamin C deficiency

D44 The following inherited diseases are associated with an increased incidence of malignancy:

A   X-linked agammaglobulinaemia
B   Beckwith–Wiedemann syndrome
C   neurofibromatosis
D   Duchenne muscular dystrophy
E   Wiskott–Aldrich syndrome

D45 The following drugs are contraindications to breast feeding:

A   daunorubicin
B   warfarin
C   atenolol
D   naproxen
E   ergotamine

D46 Amiodarone

A   prolongs the refractory period in both atria and ventricles
B   has a short half-life
C   is metabolized during first pass through the liver
D   causes microdeposits in the cornea of most patients taking the drug
E   is associated with peripheral neuropathy

D47 The following antibiotics are likely to accumulate with renal impairment:

A   metronidazole
B   erythromycin
C   benzyl penicillin
D   tobramycin
E   chlortetracycline

D48 The following drugs are highly emetic:

A cisplatin
B vincristine
C domperidone
D daunorubicin
E intrathecal methotrexate

D49 Administration of a drug

A by mouth usually results in absorption mainly from the stomach
B rectally prevents first pass metabolism
C by the sublingual route prevents first pass metabolism
D orally favours absorption of ionized molecules
E by inhalation prevents systemic side effects

D50 School refusers

A tend to leave home in the morning but do not arrive at school
B often make excuses, such as abdominal pain, for not attending school
C are typically poor achievers at school
D are disruptive when at school
E develop neurotic symptoms as adults in the majority of cases

D51 Features of infection with respiratory syncytial virus include

A purulent sputum production
B expiratory grunt
C ventilation perfusion mismatch
D permanent lung damage
E maculopapular rash

D52 Consistent features of cystic fibrosis include

A low sweat chloride
B short stature
C delayed puberty
D biliary cirrhosis
E male infertility

D53 Lung function testing in an asthmatic patient will typically show

A   a lower residual volume than in non-asthmatics
B   an increase in functional vital capacity of more than 20% after a suitable dose of nebulized salbutamol
C   a reduced diffusion capacity of carbon monoxide
D   a decreased FEV_{25-75} (forced expiratory volume between 25 and 75% of vital capacity)
E   a fall in the peak expiratory flow rate after exercising for 5 minutes

D54 Sudden infant death syndrome is more common in

✓ A   social classes IV and V
— B   Hong Kong
✓ C   winter months
— D   first born infants
⌣ E   Asians than Caucasians in the western world

D55 Projectile vomiting is characteristically associated with

— A   urinary tract infection
✓ B   occurrence immediately after feeds
✓ C   visible peristalsis
— D   anorexia
— E   acidosis

D56 The chi square test

A   can only be used on nominal data
B   can be used to test the null hypothesis that there is no difference between two samples
C   can only be applied to normal distributions
D   involves a calculation of expected values
E   involves entering the chi square table at a certain number of degrees of freedom

D57 In childhood diabetes

✓ A   diabetic retinopathy is unlikely to be found before puberty
✓ B   nephropathy may be anticipated by the presence of microalbuminuria
✓ C   lipohypertrophy is much more common than lipoatrophy
✓ D   there is an increased incidence of coeliac disease
✓ E   fructosamine can be used to monitor glycaemic control

D58 Craniopharyngioma

✓ A erodes surrounding tissues
✓ B may present as diabetes insipidus
✓ C is associated with intracranial calcification
— D responds to combination chemotherapy
— E carries a worse prognosis in older children

D59 Recognized causes of nystagmus include

✓ A congenital cataracts
✓ B phenytoin
— C warfarin
✓ D Friedreich's ataxia
✓ E neonatal intraventricular haemorrhage

D60 Bronchoconstriction is a recognized effect of

✓ A terbutaline
✓ B ibuprofen
— C nifedipine
— D paracetamol
— E digoxin

Practice examination E   Questions

E1 **Damage to the facial nerve in the internal auditory meatus will result in**

- A   drooping of the mouth
- B   decreased sensation on the ipsilateral cheek
- C   decreased sensation of taste
- D   inability to wrinkle the forehead
- E   paralysis of the lateral rectus muscle of the eye

E2 **Hypochloraemic alkalosis with hypokalaemia and low urinary chloride is seen in**

- A   congenital hypertrophic pyloric stenosis
- B   renal tubular acidosis
- C   Bartter's syndrome
- D   pseudo–Bartter's syndrome
- E   congenital chloridorrhoea

E3 **Magnesium**

- A   is primarily an extracellular cation
- B   reabsorption in the kidney is increased by parathyroid hormone
- C   levels usually fall in renal failure
- D   excess may lead to hyporeflexia
- E   toxicity may be reversed by infusion of calcium

E4 **In the fetal circulation**

- A   30% of the fetal cardiac output goes through the placenta
- B   oxygenated blood from the placenta passes through the ductus arteriosus towards the right atrium
- C   the oxygen saturation of blood in the umbilical arteries is approximately 60%
- D   blood entering the heart from the inferior vena cava is diverted directly to the left atrium via the patent foramen ovale
- E   there is one umbilical vein

E5 **Pulmonary stenosis is associated with**

- A   Noonan syndrome
- B   Turner syndrome
- C   Friedreich's ataxia
- D   Holt Oram syndrome
- E   congenital rubella

E6   Pulmonary plethora occurs with

A   transposition of the great arteries
B   Fallot's tetralogy
C   truncus arteriosus
D   total anomalous pulmonary venous drainage
E   patent ductus arteriosus

E7   In a child who is cyanosed on the second day of life, secondary to a cardiac lesion,

A   the most likely cause is total anomalous pulmonary venous drainage
B   indomethacin may help
C   there is a significant risk of bacterial endocarditis in the first month of life
D   the Pao_2 is likely to be less than 20 kPa in 100% inspired oxygen
E   there is unlikely to be evidence of heart failure

E8   Further assessment or investigation is indicated for a child who

A   demonstrates scissoring of the lower limbs at 2 weeks of age
B   appears to be left handed by the age of 1 year
C   fails to walk by the age of 16 months
D   still wets the bed at the age of four
E   has no words at the age of 1 year

E9   In the normal development of vision and fine motor function

A   infants should fix and follow a brightly coloured object through 180° by 4 weeks
B   hand to hand transfer of objects occurs from around 6 months
C   an 18-month-old child should be able to build a tower of 10 cubes
D   most 4 year olds can draw a cross
E   strabismus is unacceptable at any age

E10 In the development of the central nervous system

A ectodermal structures predominate
B neural tube closure should be complete by 6 weeks of gestation
C the cranial end of the neural tube divides into two primitive vesicles
D the cerebellum originates from the telencephalon
E motor neurons are derived from the basal plate of the spinal cord

E11 Carbon monoxide poisoning

A leads to central cyanosis
B results in a decreased arterial Po_2
C can be diagnosed several hours after death
D causes hyperventilation
E can be treated only by the administration of oxygen

E12 In the management of a child born with ambiguous genitalia

A no attempt should be made to assign a sex at the time of delivery
B the sex of rearing is determined by the karyotype, which should be ascertained urgently
C congenital adrenal hyperplasia is a diagnosis of exclusion
D cosmetic surgery should be delayed until the child is at school
E dysgenetic gonads should be removed at diagnosis

E13 Hypoglycaemia

A is rarely seen in newborn infants of diabetic mothers
B may be the sole presenting feature of growth hormone deficiency
C in diabetics is associated with ketonuria
D is less likely to lead to permanent neurological impairment in infants than older children and adults
E in an unrousable child should be corrected with a bolus of 50% dextrose

E14 Adolescents with diabetes should

A   eat a low carbohydrate diet
B   avoid strenuous exercise
C   omit their insulin dose if unable to eat because of vomiting
D   rub the injection site after administration of insulin
E   avoid a high fat diet

E15 The secretion of antidiuretic hormone is increased by

A   hypothermia
B   alcohol
C   stress
D   haemorrhage
E   cortisol

E16 Constipation may result from

A   Hirschsprung's disease
B   treatment with intramuscular pethidine
C   hypocalcaemia
D   a high milk intake
E   child abuse

E17 Bile salts

A   are formed from bilirubin
B   complex in the gut with fatty acids to form micelles
C   are essential for effective vitamin K absorption
D   undergo 50% reabsorption into the enterohepatic circulation
E   are actively reabsorbed in the distal ileum

E18 Alpha-1-antitrypsin deficiency

A   is associated with the abnormal genotype Pi MM
B   only affects homozygotes
C   can cause liver disease and pulmonary emphysema in the same patient
D   should be treated with phenobarbitone to slow the progressive hepatic dysfunction
E   can be diagnosed antenatally

E19 **The following tongue abnormalities are correctly paired with the underlying disease:**

A   fissured tongue and hypothyroidism
B   macroglossia and Beckwith–Wiedemann syndrome
C   smooth tongue and hypopituitarism
D   white tongue and scarlet fever
E   macroglossia and Down's syndrome

E20 **The following conditions or traits and their modes of inheritance are correctly paired:**

A   coeliac disease – autosomal recessive
B   blood groups A and B – autosomal dominant
C   periodic paralysis – autosomal dominant
D   Pierre Robin sequence – multifactorial
E   11β-hydroxylase deficiency – autosomal dominant

E21 **Barr bodies are present in**

A   Turner syndrome
B   normal mature oocytes
C   complete androgen insensitivity syndrome (CAIS)
D   Klinefelter syndrome
E   buccal smears from a normal female

E22 **The following are associated with fragile X syndrome:**

A   large testes
B   learning difficulties in carrier females
C   obesity
D   female distribution of secondary sexual hair
E   microcephaly

E23 **Neonatal alloimmune thrombocytopenia (NAIT)**

A   is associated with thrombocytopenia in the mother
B   results from the effects of the PlA1 antibody in the majority of cases
C   rarely presents with haemorrhagic manifestations after the first 24 h of life
D   leads to intracranial haemorrhage
E   can be prevented by a single intrauterine platelet transfusion prior to delivery

E24 Features of extravascular haemolysis include

    A   jaundice
    B   haemoglobinuria
    C   splenomegaly
    D   low reticulocyte count
    E   raised serum haptoglobin levels

E25 Red cell

    A   production is increased as a direct response to bone marrow hypoxia
    B   counts do not significantly increase for several days after entering a hypoxic atmosphere
    C   maturation is dependent on adequate vitamin A
    D   production in the neonate is almost exclusively in the bone marrow
    E   production in the shaft of the femur is insignificant by 5 years of age

E26 Features of mastocytosis include

    A   pigmented rash
    B   blister formation
    C   flushing
    D   hepatomegaly
    E   osteoporosis

E27 The following are opsonins:

    A   IgD
    B   complement
    C   C reactive protein
    D   interferon-α
    E   IgG

E28 T cell immunodeficiency is a feature of

    A   ataxia telangiectasia
    B   Wiskott–Aldrich syndrome
    C   chronic granulomatous disease
    D   Schwachmann's syndrome
    E   DiGeorge syndrome

E29 The following are recognized complications of glandular fever:

A   mouth ulceration
B   aplastic anaemia
C   nephrotic syndrome
D   transverse myelitis
E   orchitis

E30 Brucellosis

A   infection is frequently asymptomatic
B   may be transmitted by entry through human skin
C   leads to positive blood cultures in most cases
D   is usually accompanied by a neutrophil leucocytosis
E   may be complicated by suppurative lymphadenitis

E31 Human parvovirus B19

A   causes erythema infectiosum
B   is no longer infectious when the rash appears
C   may cause aplastic crises in children with hereditary
     spherocytosis
D   infection during pregnancy can cause anencephaly
E   can cause hydrops fetalis

E32 The following are characteristics of falciparum malaria:

A   transmission by the male *Anopheles* mosquito
B   a latent hepatic stage
C   some resistance in patients with glucose-6-phosphatase
     deficiency
D   massive splenomegaly
E   a fever recurring every third day

E33 Polyarticular onset juvenile chronic arthritis

A   has a female predominance
B   carries a worse prognosis if IgM rheumatoid factor is
     positive
C   rarely involves the cervical spine
D   is frequently associated with iridocyclitis
E   has a characteristic butterfly rash over the bridge of the
     nose

E34 Surfactant

A   is produced by the alveolar type I epithelial cell
B   is not detectable in the lung before 32 weeks' gestation
C   increases the surface tension in alveoli
D   deficiency can only be treated with general supportive measures
E   production is impaired in an environment with a pH < 7.25

E35 Neonatal convulsions may be caused by

A   hypomagnesaemia
B   hyperkalaemia
C   pyridoxine dependency
D   cephalhaematoma
E   herpes simplex virus infection

E36 Necrotizing enterocolitis is associated with

A   epidemics
B   thrombocytopenia
C   malabsorption
D   bile-stained aspirates
E   air in the portal tree on abdominal X-ray

E37 Pulmonary hypoplasia is a consequence of

A   congenital varicella zoster
B   anencephaly
C   posterior urethral valves
D   congenital diaphragmatic hernia
E   exomphalos

E38 Proteinuria

A   may result from the loss of cationic charge in the glomerular basement membrane
B   is more common on waking than in the evening
C   is a late sign of diabetic nephropathy
D   is a feature of Wilson's disease
E   may be quantified in childhood from a single specimen of urine

E39 Impaired renal function in the presence of normal-sized kidneys on ultrasound is consistent with

A vesicoureteric reflux
B polycystic kidneys
C minimal change nephrotic syndrome
D Wilms' tumour
E haemolytic uraemic syndrome

E40 Recognized findings on the electroencephalogram (EEG) include

A a reduction in high frequency (α and β) rhythms with increasing maturity
B hypsarrhythmia in infants with tuberous sclerosis
C generalized slow wave activity in the presence of a cerebral abscess
D a 3 Hz spike and wave pattern associated with structural abnormalities of the brain
E a burst suppression pattern following severe perinatal asphyxia

E41 Cerebral blood flow

A represents about 15% of the resting cardiac output
B is highly susceptible to changes in systemic blood pressure
C increases in response to hypocapnia
D is highly dependent on sympathetic nervous control
E increases in response to severe hypoxia

E42 Vitamin A deficiency

A is associated with xerophthalmia
B is common in children with coeliac disease
C is commonly found in patients in the cystic fibrosis clinic
D in pregnant women causes neural tube defects in the fetus
E can be treated with halibut liver oil

E43 Wilms' tumours occur more commonly in children

A with aniridia
B with Beckwith–Wiedemann syndrome
C of the male sex
D with a family history of nephroblastoma
E who have a mother with systemic lupus erythematosus

E44 A bitemporal hemianopia may be caused by

A papilloedema
B occipital lobe infarction
C pituitary adenoma
D suprasellar meningioma
E aneurysm of the posterior cerebral artery

E45 Symptoms of drug withdrawal in the neonate may follow maternal use of

A methadone
B temazepam
C paracetamol
D cannabis
E lithium

E46 Nitric oxide

A is synthesized in endothelial cells from the amino acid lysine
B production is stimulated by acetylcholine
C is an inflammatory mediator
D may be of benefit in the treatment of adult respiratory distress syndrome (ARDS)
E combines with haemoglobin to form methaemoglobin

E47 The following are recognized treatments of hyperkalaemia:

A intravenous salbutamol
B oral calcium resonium
C oral sodium polystyrene sulphonate
D infusion of glucose and insulin
E sodium dihydrogen phosphate

E48 Beta-antagonists may cause

A heart failure
B increased airway resistance
C hyperglycaemia
D bradycardia in newborn infants of mothers receiving the drug
E psychosis

E49 Warfarin

A   is teratogenic
B   is antagonized by protamine
C   action is potentiated by barbiturates
D   activity is decreased by erythromycin
E   may precipitate glucose intolerance

E50 Schizophrenia in adolescence

A   may be familial
B   presents insidiously
C   is usually associated with distinctive abnormal behavioural patterns in childhood
D   may be difficult to differentiate clinically from drug-induced states
E   should be managed without neuroleptic treatment

E51 In the management of asthma

A   inhaled powder devices are inappropriate for use by children under the age of 8 years
B   delivery of inhaled steroid to the bronchial tree is improved by use of a spacer device in children of all ages
C   there is no place for sodium cromoglycate as prophylaxis in children with daily symptoms
D   short stature is a well recognized complication of treatment with low-dose inhaled corticosteroids
E   peak expiratory flow rate should be monitored from the age of three in children on prophylactic medication

E52 Causes of bronchiectasis include

A   whooping cough
B   chicken pox
C   cystic fibrosis
D   foreign body inhalation
E   Williams–Campbell syndrome

E53 The administration of 100% oxygen

A   leads to tachycardia
B   decreases cardiac output
C   decreases pulmonary vascular resistance
D   increases glucose utilization
E   causes atelectasis

E54 There is an increased incidence of pneumothorax in patients with

A   pulmonary tuberculosis
B   staphylococcal pneumonia
C   Ehlers–Danlos syndrome
D   asthma
E   *Bordetella pertussis* infection

E55 Neck stiffness occurs in

A   cerebral palsy
B   fibrodysplasia ossificans (myositis ossificans)
C   poliomyelitis
D   metoclopramide use
E   salicylate overdose

E56 The following statements about the normal distribution are true:

A   it is fully characterized by its mean and variance
B   the median is greater than the mean
C   the data are non-parametric
D   96% of the population lies within one standard deviation of the mean
E   it may be used to approximate the binomial distribution

E57 Hypertension is a feature of

A   phaeochromocytoma
B   renal vein thrombosis
C   Down's syndrome
D   treatment with diazoxide
E   porphyria

E58 Causes of generalized hypotonia in a 3-month-old infant include

A   cerebral palsy
B   Werdnig–Hoffmann syndrome
C   peroneal muscular atrophy
D   myasthenia gravis
E   Duchenne muscular dystrophy

E59 The following are typical features of obsessive compulsive neurosis:

A ruminations
B passivity feelings
C repetitive handwashing
D lack of insight
E olfactory hallucinations

E60 A young woman with phenylketonuria (PKU) wishes to start a family.

A Half of her offspring are statistically likely to have the disease
B She must start a phenylalanine restricted diet prior to conception
C The fetus is at an increased risk of microcephaly
D Cord blood phenylalanine levels can be used to indicate whether the baby has PKU
E She has a deficiency of phenylalanine hydroxylase

Practice examination A   Answers

A1 FTFTF
The 1st and 2nd sacral nerves provide the motor supply for plantar flexion of the foot, and the ankle jerk. The sensory supply for the sole of the foot comes from the 1st sacral root. Penile erection and detrusor muscle contraction are parasympathetic functions supplied by the sacral outflow, in contrast to ejaculation and detrusor relaxation, supplied by the sympathetic nervous system, via the thoracolumbar outflow.

A2 TFTFT
Teeth have enamel, dentine, cementum and pulp. The main body of the tooth is composed of dentine which has a strong bony structure. It is made of hydroxyapatite crystals in a collagen meshwork. The dentine is covered by a layer of enamel which is extremely hard and is resistant to acids, enzymes and other corrosive agents. The enamel is formed prior to eruption of the tooth. Cementum is a bony substance which lines the tooth socket and pulp is at the centre of the tooth and is composed of connective tissue, nerves, blood vessels and lymphatics. There are 20 deciduous teeth and 32 permanent teeth.

A3 FTTTF
Enzymatic defects at any stage of the urea cycle result in high blood urea. Examples include ornithine transcarbamylase deficiency or N-acetylglutamate synthetase deficiency. Patients with severe defects present in the neonatal period with coma and acute metabolic crisis. With less severe mutations symptoms may not present until precipitated by a high protein intake, an intercurrent infection or period of dehydration. Other causes of hyperammonaemia include liver disease, Reye's syndrome, lactic acidosis, the ketotic hyperglycinaemias and ureterostomy. Raised ammonia is not a feature of burns, in which metabolic disturbances result from tissue catabolism and hypovolaemia, or of acute renal failure.

A4 FTTFF
In metabolic acidosis the pH is low, the hydrogen ion concentration is high, the bicarbonate is low and there is a base deficit (i.e. negative value of the base excess). In metabolic alkalosis, such as in pyloric stenosis or following severe vomiting from another cause, the pH is raised, the hydrogen ion concentration is reduced, the bicarbonate is high and the base excess has a positive value. The renal compensation of respiratory acidosis also results in a positive base excess.

A5 FTTTF

Causes of electromechanical dissociation include hypoxaemia, severe acidosis, hypovolaemia, hyperkalaemia, tension pneumothorax, pericardial tamponade and overdoses of β-blockers, tricyclic antidepressants and calcium channel blocking drugs. The outcome is poor unless the cause is identified and treated. In the meantime, cardiac massage, adrenaline and ventilation in 100% oxygen should be administered.

A6 FTTFF

Infants with Fallot's tetralogy are not usually cyanosed at birth. Cyanosis develops in most by the end of the first year of life. Pulmonary atresia with or without an intact septum usually presents with cyanosis shortly after birth. Coarctation usually presents with cardiac failure. Endocardial fibroelastosis is a cardiomyopathy of unknown aetiology. There is diffuse thickening of the endocardium and the dilated chambers contract poorly. Most babies present with cardiac failure within the first 3 months of life.

A7 FTTTF

During inspiration the negative thoracic pressure is transmitted to the veins of the chest and the central venous pressure falls. The 'a' wave is prominent when right ventricular hypertrophy leads to increased resistance to filling, for example, in pulmonary stenosis or pulmonary hypertension. In complete heart block (complete atrioventricular dissociation) regular 'a' waves occur but they are dissociated from the arterial pulsation.

A8 TFTTF

Dermatitis herpetiformis is a variant of coeliac disease and manifests as an itchy blistering rash on elbows, knees, shoulders and buttocks, associated with a gluten sensitive enteropathy. The characteristic skin lesions in neurofibromatosis are café-au-lait patches and fibromata. Most cases of erythema multiforme follow infection with viruses or mycoplasma and treatment with various drugs, including sulphonamides. Kasabach–Merritt syndrome is the association of thrombocytopenia with large cavernous haemangiomata or diffuse haemangiomatosis. Pyoderma gangrenosum is seen in a minority of cases of Crohn's disease and ulcerative colitis.

A9 TFFTT

A normal 2 year old would be expected to go upstairs alone and down, holding on, two feet per step, to build a tower of six or seven cubes, and imitate a vertical stroke with a pencil. Two year olds are generally dry by day. This is sometimes given as the age for dryness at night, if lifted out late in the evening, but the age range for this milestone is wide. In practice it would be more realistic to expect dryness at night by the age of three. Speech is limited to two or three word phrases, whereas the ability to converse takes until at least the age of three. Recognition of colours is not usually seen until the age of three, although colour matching may happen earlier.

A10 TFTTF
A child may have a large head simply because of a familial tendency. Pathological causes include hydrocephalus, subdural effusions, cerebral tumours, megalencephaly and hydranencephaly. An infant with achondroplasia has a big head because of megalencephaly and slight ventricular enlargement. In Russell–Silver syndrome there is dwarfism with a large head. Craniosynostosis causes an abnormally shaped head, as a result of premature closure of the cranial sutures. A child with Down's syndrome has a small brachycephalic head.

A11 TTFFF
The lining of the gut and its derivatives, including liver and pancreas, are of endodermal origin, whereas the mesodermal germ layer gives rise to muscular components and the peritoneum. The ectoderm contributes the anal pit, which forms the distal part of the anal canal. Structures from the oesophagus to the point of entry of the bile duct into the duodenum arise from the foregut and the hindgut gives rise to the large gut from the distal third of the transverse colon. The midgut, which is temporarily connected to the yolk sac by means of the vitelline duct, forms the structures in between. The intestinal loop rotates around the superior mesenteric artery through 270° counterclockwise and failure leads to either malfixation or malrotation. The cloacal membrane divides into the anterior urogenital membrane and posterior anal membrane. Failure of the latter to rupture, either alone or in combination with failed development of the anal pit, leads to varying degrees of anal atresia.

A12 FTTFF
A 5.0–5.5 ET tube would be most appropriate (formula: internal diameter = age/4 + 4). Defibrillation should start at 2 × weight (Joules). Initial fluid replacement with colloid for hypovolaemic shock should be at least 10 × weight (ml).

A13 FTFTF

Gonadal development is abnormal in Turner syndrome, leading to infertility in most cases, but the female external genitalia are not ambiguous. In congenital adrenal hyperplasia, both males and females are virilized, leading to ambiguity in the females. Rarer forms may lead to incomplete virilization of males. Micropenis may be found in males with panhypopituitarism, due to gonadotrophin deficiency, but in other respects the morphology of external genitalia is unambiguous. 5α-Reductase catalyses the conversion of testosterone to dihydrotestosterone (DHT), required for the development of external genitalia. Deficiency does not affect development of Wolffian (internal) structures or spermatogenesis. In androgen insensitivity syndromes there is an abnormal response to normal production of testosterone. Partial androgen insensitivity syndrome (PAIS) generally presents with ambiguous genitalia but, in CAIS (formerly testicular feminization), the genitalia are phenotypically female. These patients usually present with bilateral inguinal herniae or primary amenorrhoea.

A14 FFTFT

Disproportionate short stature results from disorders affecting the long bones and spine to a differing extent. Dyschondroplasias, including achondroplasia and hypochondroplasia, result in short limbs for spine, whereas the mucopolysaccharidoses (Hurler, Hunter, Morquio but not Sanfilippo syndromes) result in a short spine compared to the limbs. Most other causes of short stature do not lead to disproportion. They include chromosomal abnormalities, endocrine disorders such as hypothyroidism, growth hormone deficiency, Cushing's disease and panhypopituitarism, metabolic disorders, poor nutrition and any chronic disease process. Septo-optic dysplasia (de Morsier's syndrome) leads to panhypopituitarism, in addition to central neurological deficits. Untreated precocious puberty causes premature epiphyseal fusion.

A15 FFTTT

In patients with anorexia nervosa, there is an immature secretory pattern for luteinizing hormone (LH), resulting in amenorrhoea or delay of pubertal development. Growth hormone responses to stimulation are blunted although basal levels are raised and somatomedin levels are low. Overall cortisol production is not affected but levels are raised due to reduced clearance and the normal diurnal variation in levels is lost. Tri-iodothyronine (T3) is usually reduced, thyroxine normal and thyroid stimulating hormone low or normal. Hypokalaemia and alkalosis may result from vomiting and laxative abuse. Irreversible hypoglycaemia, hypothermia and secondary infection are the most common terminal events in the 5% of cases who die as a result of their condition.

A16 TTFTT
The causes of non-infective diarrhoea are numerous and include Hirschsprung's disease (which is more likely to present with constipation) and other surgical conditions, malabsorption including abetalipoproteinaemia, allergy, immune deficiency, autoimmune diseases, chronic inflammatory bowel disease, metabolic disorders including hypocalcaemia and hyperthyroidism, drugs and radiotherapy. Hypothyroidism is a cause of constipation.

A17 TFFTF
All neonates with jaundice persisting beyond 10 days should be investigated. The majority of patients will have an unconjugated hyperbilirubinaemia (unconjugated more than 70% of total). Causes of prolonged unconjugated neonatal jaundice include breast milk jaundice, hypothyroidism, intestinal stasis causing increased enterohepatic circulation (e.g. Hirschsprung's disease, pyloric stenosis, meconium ileus), haemolytic causes, Gilbert's syndrome and Crigler–Najjar syndrome. Conjugated hyperbilirubinaemia is an indication of intrahepatic or extrahepatic cholestasis. Causes of this include biliary atresia, choledochal cyst, alpha-1-antitrypsin deficiency, galactosaemia, fructosaemia, mucopolysaccharidosis, a complication of parenteral nutrition, Dubin–Johnson syndrome and Rotor syndrome. Some diseases can present with conjugated or unconjugated jaundice and include viral hepatitis, cystic fibrosis, sepsis and congenital infections.

A18 TFTFT
Iron is absorbed from the proximal small intestine, especially the duodenum. Its absorption is increased by ascorbic acid or the presence of iron deficiency. Antacids bind to iron, impairing absorption. Ferrous salts are more efficiently absorbed from the small intestine than ferric salts.

A19 TFFTF
Recurrent abdominal pain occurs in approximately 10% of school children and an organic disorder is demonstrated in only 10% of these. Two-thirds have associated vomiting, half have pallor

during the attack and one in five have headaches. A family history of recurrent abdominal pain is common. Pain away from the umbilicus is more likely to be organic. Non-organic pain may be colicky, continuous, aching or sharp. It may occur by day or night but if it wakes the child at night the clinician should be alerted to the possibility of an organic cause. Although rare, the acute porphyrias are recognized causes of abdominal pain with or without vomiting. Menstruation may present without bleeding in cases of imperforate hymen, leading to haematocolpos.

A20 FTTFF
Galactosaemia is an autosomal recessive condition; note that metabolic disorders are more likely to be recessive than dominant. Neural tube disorders show multifactorial inheritance and inheritance of Fabry disease is X-linked recessive.

A21 TTFTT
Clinical features of Prader–Willi syndrome include hypotonia, short stature and obesity, hypogonadism, intellectual impairment, characteristic facies, high incidence of diabetes mellitus, squint, scoliosis, and small hands and feet. In the first year of life, hypotonia and feeding difficulties may lead to failure to thrive. Genetics is complicated and closely related to Angelman syndrome. Both are associated with interstitial deletions in the same region of the long arm of chromosome 15, identified in around 70% of cases. A smaller proportion of cases display uniparental disomy where two copies of a chromosome pair are inherited from one parent and none from the other. In Prader–Willi syndrome, DNA studies have shown the cases of deletion to be paternally inherited, whereas cases of uniparental disomy are maternally inherited. These findings suggest that the phenotype of Prader–Willi results from failure to inherit the critical region of the paternal chromosome 15. In the case of Angelman syndrome, deletions are maternal and uniparental disomy occurs less frequently.

A22 TFTTT
The normal human karyotype consists of a total of 46 chromosomes, comprising the two sex chromosomes and 22 pairs of autosomes, numbered from 1 to 22, in order of decreasing size. The centromere separates short (p) and long (q) arms on all chromosomes. Apart from size and centromere position, chromosomes are distinguished from one another by characteristic banding patterns shown up by staining with Giemsa, hence the process is known as G-banding. The Philadelphia chromosome is

the result of a translocation between chromosomes 9 and 22. It occurs in most cases of chronic myeloid leukaemia and about 25% cases of adult acute lymphoblastic leukaemia (ALL); its presence in childhood ALL is a poor prognostic sign. Cri du chat syndrome is characterized by microcephaly, micrognathia, downward (anti-Mongoloid) slanting palpebral fissures, a hypoplastic larynx and severe intellectual retardation.

A23 TTFFT
The most common cause of eosinophilia is atopic disease. Any of the parasitic diseases may also lead to raised counts, as may non-eczematous skin disorders including psoriasis, pemphigus and dermatitis herpetiformis. Drug sensitivity, lymphomas, pulmonary eosinophilia, polyarteritis nodosa, eosinophilic leukaemia and recovery from acute infections or chemotherapy are also recognized causes. Tuberculosis leads to a monocytosis and steroids stimulate neutrophil production.

A24 TFFFT
G6PD deficiency is an X-linked disorder of the red cell, leading to haemolytic anaemia in response to certain infections, ingestion of fava beans (in the Mediterranean variety of the disorder) and exposure to oxidant drugs. Drugs to avoid include salicylates, most antimalarials, sulphonamides, nalidixic acid, nitrofurantoin and chloramphenicol. Any cause of haemolytic anaemia may predispose to the development of pigment gallstones. The direct Coombs' test detects complement or antibody on the surface of red cells and is therefore a test for immune haemolytic anaemia.

A25 FFTFF
Loss of splenic function may result from congenital asplenia, splenectomy or total body irradiation. Sickle cell disease is associated with a large spleen in infancy and early childhood which diminishes in size in the course of childhood due to infarction (autosplenectomy). Patients with hyposplenism are particularly prone to infection with encapsulated organisms, including *Pneumococcus* and *Haemophilus influenzae* type B.

A26 TTFTF
The bleeding time is an *in vivo* test of platelet and capillary function. Idiopathic thrombocytopenic purpura, hypersplenism and haemolytic uraemic syndrome all cause thrombocytopenia and uraemia, von Willebrand's disease and aspirin treatment affect platelet function. The bleeding time is sometimes prolonged

in Henoch–Schönlein purpura and connective tissue disorders, where the platelet count is normal but there is increased capillary permeability resulting in purpura.

A27 FTFFT

Isolated IgA deficiency is the most common primary immunodeficiency. Most individuals remain asymptomatic, and those with recurrent infections tend to improve with age. Minor recurrent sinopulmonary infections are the most common complications in childhood. However, severe pneumonia and troublesome ear infections can occur. Infections at other sites are relatively rare and include an increased incidence of *Giardia* infection of the gut. Allergic disease occurs with an increased frequency in patients with immune deficiency and particularly with selective IgA deficiency. Autoimmune disorders are also more common in these patients. Usual treatment of IgA deficiency is to commence antibiotic treatment early in the course of an infection but some patients require long-term antibiotic prophylaxis. Hereditary angio-oedema is due to deficiency of the complement control protein, C1 esterase inhibitor, resulting in spontaneous episodes of localized oedema.

A28 FTFTF

Live vaccines should not be given in the following circumstances: patients who have received chemotherapy or radiation within the last year, patients with a malignant disorder such as leukaemia or lymphoma, with immunosuppressive disorders, those receiving high dose corticosteroids or patients who have received immunoglobulin within the last 3 months. Immunoglobulin may, however, be given simultaneously with live vaccines if indicated. It is appropriate to give a live vaccine in the following circumstances: non-febrile common cold, antibiotic treatment, previous history of the infection, stable neurological conditions. If a patient has an acute illness the vaccination should be postponed until the fever has resolved.

A29 FTTTF

Staphylococcus aureus is the most common organism cultured from blood or pus in bacterial bone and joint infections at all ages. Ritter's disease, also known as staphylococcal scalded skin syndrome, toxic epidermal necrolysis and Lyell's syndrome, is caused by the toxin from *Staphylococcus aureus*, phage type 71. Coagulase negative staphylococci are the organisms usually involved in the colonization of ventriculoperitoneal shunts but *Staph. aureus*, streptococci and coliforms are occasionally seen.

Erythema toxicum is a common, benign, self-limiting, erythematous reaction seen in the first few days of life. It consists of erythema with eosinophilic pustules and papules over the face, trunk and limbs, and is not an infective condition.

A30 FFTTT
The incubation period of rubella is 14–18 days. It is characteristically a mild illness, relatively free from complications, except when infection occurs in the first trimester of pregnancy. Polyarthritis, encephalitis and myelitis may all follow infection with rubella, but the outlook is generally good.

A31 TFFTT
Lyme disease is a multisystem disorder which consists of a prodromal febrile illness with a rash known as erythema chronicum migrans. Without antibiotic treatment many patients will develop the late manifestations of the disease which may be cardiac, neurological or rheumatological. Cardiac involvement is typically myocarditis, left ventricular dysfunction and atrioventricular block. ELISA of specific IgM or IgG antibodies may be used to confirm the diagnosis although they are associated with both false positive and negative results. Tetracycline is the drug of choice for older children, and phenoxymethylpenicillin or erythromycin for younger patients. Cefotaxime or penicillin are used once later manifestations have developed.

A32 TTTFF
ABO incompatibility leads to unconjugated hyperbilirubinaemia from day one of life due to haemolysis. Group A, B and O mothers have IgM isoagglutinins which do not cross the placenta but 10% of group O women have IgG anti-A (rarely anti-B) which will haemolyse the red cells of a group A (rarely B) infant. Since these antibodies are present before pregnancy, all pregnancies, including the first, are equally at risk, unlike in Rhesus incompatibility, where the risk increases progressively. The direct Coombs' test is negative or weakly positive and the jaundice usually responds to hydration and phototherapy, rarely requiring exchange transfusion. ABO incompatibility may protect against the effects of Rhesus incompatibility by removing fetal red cells from the maternal circulation before a significant response is raised to the fetal Rhesus antigen. A direct (conjugated) bilirubin of more than 30 μmol/l or 15% of the total bilirubin is abnormal and a direct level as high as 100 μmol/l is strongly suggestive of an obstructive cause or hepatitis.

A33 FTTFF
Any baby born dead after 28 weeks' gestation is classified as a stillbirth. All live births, irrespective of gestation or duration of life, must be registered by the Registrar of Births, Marriages and Deaths. The perinatal mortality rate includes deaths of live births at less than 7 days of age and stillbirths. The neonatal mortality rate includes deaths at less than 28 days and excludes stillbirths. It is sometimes subdivided into early (0–6 days) and late (7–27 days) neonatal mortality. Infant mortality includes all deaths up to 1 year after live birth and is equivalent to the sum of neonatal and postneonatal (28 days–1 year) mortality rates. All of the mortality rates are expressed as a number per 1000 livebirths (or livebirths plus stillbirths in the case of perinatal mortality) and age at death is not corrected for gestational age. Low birthweight infants account for approximately 50% of all infant deaths in developed countries (figures from International Collaborative Effort).

A34 TFFTT
Measurement of maternal α-fetoprotein is undertaken at 16–20 weeks' gestation. Causes of elevated levels include anencephaly, open spina bifida, anterior abdominal wall defects, congenital nephrotic syndrome, multiple pregnancies and placental haemangioma. The level of α-fetoprotein in maternal serum tends to be lower in pregnancies with trisomy 21.

A35 TTFFF
Bronchopulmonary dysplasia (BPD) is a chronic lung disease in babies who have required mechanical ventilation. It is characterized by hypoxia, hypercapnia and oxygen dependence. Oxygen therapy should maintain oxygen saturations above 90% to prevent pulmonary hypertension. Hypercapnia may be acceptable to aid weaning from the ventilator if the baby is not acidotic and is otherwise well. The chest X-ray shows hyperexpanded lung fields with focal areas of opacification and cysts. Mortality of babies with severe BPD is 30%. Surviving babies require frequent hospital admissions with lower respiratory tract infections and are at risk of developing right sided heart failure. They often fail to thrive (30%) and many have developmental delay (30%). There is an increased incidence of sudden infant death syndrome.

A36 FTFFT
Fully breast fed babies have loose stools which may contain curd and may be bright green in colour. They may be frequent, with

up to 20 stools in 24 h, or as infrequent as every 4 days or so. Ninety per cent of babies pass meconium within the first 24 h of life and delay may be due to Hirschsprung's disease, a meconium plug or other causes of intestinal obstruction. When a newborn baby has blood in the stool it is essential to determine whether it is swallowed maternal blood, from the delivery or a cracked nipple, or from the baby, which may indicate haemorrhagic disease of the newborn.

A37 TTTFT
Membranous nephropathy or glomerulonephritis may be seen in association with hepatitis B, systemic lupus erythematosus (SLE), drug treatment with gold or penicillamine and some malignancies of the bowel and bronchus. It presents mainly in adults, predominantly in males, with nephrotic syndrome and spontaneously remits in approximately 30% of cases. The remainder eventually progress to chronic renal failure. Biopsy reveals diffuse thickening of the glomerular basement membrane with immune complex deposition, whereas proliferation is seen in postinfectious and crescentic glomerulonephritis.

A38 FFTFT
HUS is characterized by microangiopathic haemolytic anaemia, thrombocytopenia and acute renal failure. It typically affects infants and young children in epidemics usually with a diarrhoeal prodrome. Older children have an atypical sporadic variety which may have a respiratory prodrome. The most important aspects of treatment are early correction of the anaemia by blood transfusions, detailed attention to fluid balance and treatment of the renal failure, if necessary by dialysis. Treatment of the diarrhoea with antibiotics is of no proven benefit and may, in some cases, worsen the disease by precipitating further toxin release. Hypertension, if present, is usually mild, although sporadic HUS in older children may be associated with severe hypertension. (See also C39.)

A39 FFTTF
This autosomal recessive disease presents with massive bilateral renal enlargement which may be sufficient to obstruct normal labour. Maternal oligohydramnios due to poor production of urine sometimes leads to Potter's syndrome. Prognosis is generally very poor, initial outcome depending on pulmonary status and the degree of renal function. The infantile form of polycystic disease is associated with hepatic fibrosis which may lead to portal

hypertension. Adult polycystic disease is autosomal dominant. Although small cysts are sometimes detectable at birth on ultra-sound scanning, signs and symptoms, such as hypertension and haematuria, do not usually occur until later in life.

A40 FTTTF

Subdural effusions may occur following bacterial meningitis, particularly in infancy. Seizures occur in 20–30% of children, most within the first 48–72 h in hospital, but epilepsy may be a long-term complication. Sensorineural deafness is the commonest long-term complication of meningitis. Inappropriate secretion of anti-diuretic hormone may occur in the acute phase, but diabetes insipidus is not recognized.

A41 FTTTT

Benign intracranial hypertension is a syndrome of symptomatic raised intracranial pressure, with headache, nausea and vomiting. Visual symptoms are occasionally present and papilloedema may be unilateral or bilateral. In other respects, the patient is neuro-logically intact and cerebrospinal fluid analysis is normal. The cause is unknown in up to half of cases. Obesity, head injury, various endocrinological and haematological disorders, drugs and infections make up most of the remainder. The diagnosis of benign intracranial hypertension is sometimes made in patients with venous sinus thrombosis, which is clearly not a very benign condition. Given that benign intracranial hypertension can also lead to permanent optic nerve damage, the term 'benign' should be treated with caution.

A42 TTFTF

Infantile spasms are an uncommon type of seizure and the overall prognosis in terms of subsequent epilepsy and developmental delay is poor. They start most commonly between the ages of 3 and 8 months. A family history is very uncommon unless there is an inherited cause such as tuberous sclerosis. The spasms are often resistant to therapy but ACTH or benzodiazepines are sometimes of benefit.

A43 TFTFF

Kwashiorkor typically arises when a breast fed child is weaned onto a diet which is low in protein. Oedema is associated with a low serum albumin but it is due to dietary deficiency. The main pathological features are atrophy of the pancreas and gut mucosa resulting in malabsorption. Skin changes include pigmentation, desquamation and ulceration. The legs, buttocks and perineum are most commonly involved in contrast to pellagra in which the changes occur mainly on the exposed skin. The widely accepted Wellcome classification of protein energy deficiency is as follows:

A   Marasmus: weight less than 60% of Boston median for age
B   Marasmic kwashiorkor: weight below 60%. Oedema present
C   Kwashiorkor: weight more than 60%. Oedema present
D   Underweight: weight 60–80%. No oedema.

(80% of the Boston median weight for age is about the 3rd centile.)

A44 FTTFF
The differential diagnosis of anterior mediastinal masses includes lymphoma, germ cell tumour, rhabdomyosarcoma, Ewing's sarcoma and thymoma, which are all malignant, and teratoma, cystic hygroma, haemangioma and thymic cyst, which are benign. The malignant tumours neuroblastoma, ganglioneuroblastoma, sarcoma and phaeochromocytoma and benign ganglioneuroma, Schwann cell tumour, neurofibroma and bronchogenic cyst, may all present in the posterior mediastinum.

A45 TFTTT
Seventy-five per cent of children with Down's syndrome have small lens opacities and developmental cataracts are seen in infants with galactosaemia and Lowe's (oculocerebrorenal) syndrome. They are also found in infants with congenital infections including toxoplasmosis but not cytomegalovirus. Diabetic cataract is rare and occurs in poorly controlled diabetics, associated with osmotic changes in the lens.

A46 TFTTT
A solution of 8.4% sodium bicarbonate contains 1000 mmol/l sodium, compared with 140 mmol/l in serum and 150 mmol/l in normal saline solutions. A fall in hydrogen ion concentration following bicarbonate infusion leads to intracellular shift of potassium and increased binding of calcium to serum proteins with the effect of reducing plasma ionized calcium. Carbon dioxide, which passes readily into cells and the CSF, rises transiently following administration of bicarbonate, causing transient acidosis. The oxyhaemoglobin dissociation curve is displaced to the left, thus reducing oxygen delivery to the tissues.

A47 FTFFT
Cisapride stimulates gastrointestinal motility by increasing tone in
the lower oesophageal sphincter, accelerating gastric emptying
and decreasing colonic transit time. It is thought to increase
release of acetylcholine in the gut wall, but has no antidopamin-
ergic or direct parasympathomimetic effect. It undergoes extensive first pass metabolism, the products of which are excreted in
the urine and faeces. Side effects include abdominal cramps and
diarrhoea, and occasional headaches, seizures, extrapyramidal
disturbance and tachycardia. There is also a recognized risk of
ventricular arrhythmias associated with the simultaneous administration of imidazole antifungals and any conditions or treatment
leading to the prolongation of the QT interval.

A48 FTFFF
Approximately 5% of patients allergic to aspirin are also sensitive
to paracetamol. Paracetamol is metabolized in the liver resulting
in a toxic metabolite which is normally inactivated by conjugation
to glutathione. With overdoses the supply of glutathione becomes
depleted and the toxic metabolite combines instead with hepatic
cell membranes leading to centrilobular necrosis. *N*-acetylcysteine
administered by infusion over 20 h protects the liver, possibly by
restoring levels of glutathione or by acting as an alternative
substrate for the toxic metabolites. The prothombin time is the
best guide to the severity of the damage, liver enzyme assays
being poor indicators.

A49 TTFFF
H_2-antagonists, of which cimetidine and ranitidine are the most
widely used, are competitive antagonists of the actions of histamine on H_2-receptors. H_2-receptors are present throughout the
body, but the major clinical benefit is the competitive antagonism
of receptors on gastric parietal cells so inhibiting gastric acid
secretion. Cimetidine readily crosses lipid barriers such as the
blood–brain barrier and placenta, ranitidine less so. They have no
significant effect on gastric emptying time, lower oesophageal
tone or pancreatic secretions.

A50 TFFFT
Bulimia nervosa comprises preoccupation with food and a phobic
fear of fatness, leading to binges of eating and measures, such as
self-induced vomiting and laxative use, to counteract the fatten-
ing effects of the binges. The abnormal eating pattern, rather than
weight loss is the hallmark of bulimia, although the vomiting and

purgation may lead to physical side effects including hypokalaemia and impaired renal function, cardiac arrhythmias and pitting of the teeth from gastric acid. Menstrual disturbances are relatively rare, compared with anorexia nervosa, and the weight is usually normal. The onset is generally in older adolescence or adulthood and there may be a past history of anorexia nervosa.

A51 FTTFT
Mycoplasma is a very unlikely cause of focal consolidation with effusion, which is more likely to be seen in *Strep. pneumoniae* infection. Respiratory involvement of mycoplasma is more commonly manifest as mild upper respiratory tract infection, bronchitis, bronchiolitis or bronchopneumonia. Compression collapse of the underlying lung is inevitable with an effusion. If the compressed lung is otherwise normal, a large effusion may cause mediastinal shift away from the affected side. However, the disease process underlying the effusion may in itself lead to further substantial collapse, more than could be accounted for by compression alone. In this situation, mediastinal shift may be towards the affected side. Chylous effusions may result from obstruction of the thoracic duct. Effusions with a high protein content and lymphocyte predominance are seen in tuberculosis.

A52 TFFTF
The sweat test remains the major diagnostic tool for the confirmation of CF. It is usually delayed until the infant reaches 4 weeks and at least 3 kg; younger, smaller infants tend to produce insufficient sweat. At least 100 mg of sweat should be obtained by pilocarpine iontophoresis. Sodium and chloride concentrations of more than 70 mmol/l are definitely abnormal and indicative of CF, values of less than 50 mmol/l are normal and values between 50 and 70 mmol/l are equivocal and require further consideration. Dry skin at any age produces small sweat volumes and may give falsely raised sweat levels. Repeated studies have confirmed that high levels of sweat sodium are found in 98–99% of CF homozygotes.

A53 TFFFT
Infants with asthma commonly wheeze with viral infections but have long symptom free periods in between. An episodic night cough, even in the absence of wheeze, is another common pattern. A monophonic wheeze is suggestive of obstruction in a single large airway, whereas the polyphonic wheeze of multiple small

and medium sized airways is characteristic of asthma. Almost all 5 and 6 year olds with asthma are atopic and negative skin test results would therefore put some doubt on the diagnosis. Localized change on the chest X-ray suggests the possibility of an alternative diagnosis, but segmental or lobar atelectasis is common in asthma due to mucus plugging.

A54 FTTFT
The atmospheric pressure decreases progressively with increasing altitude (e.g. 760 mmHg at sea level but 523 mmHg at 3300 m), while the concentration of oxygen remains constant (21%). This results in a decrease in the partial pressure of oxygen from 159 mmHg (21% × 760 mmHg) at sea level to 110 mmHg (21% × 523 mmHg) at 3300 m. Responses to high altitude include hyperventilation, polycythaemia, a shift of the oxyhaemoglobin dissociation curve to the right secondary to an increase in 2,3-diphosphoglycerate, an increased number of mitochondria and oxidative enzymes and an increase in cardiac output. Pulmonary vasoconstriction occurs in response to alveolar hypoxia and right ventricular hypertrophy may result.

A55 TFFTF
Long bone fractures are generally difficult to attribute to non-accidental injury (NAI) but spiral fractures are strongly suggestive. Posterior rib fractures in otherwise healthy children are usually due to NAI, as a result of compression or kicking. Anterior fractures are more likely to be accidental, especially if single. Of all skull fractures, a linear fracture of the parietal bone is the most likely to be innocent in origin. NAI is more likely the further away from the parietal bone the fractures are found and if they are more than 5 mm wide, multiple, complex, depressed or growing. Metaphyseal fractures are caused by avulsion from shaking. Clavicular fractures are common in abused children with multiple fractures but in themselves are not sufficient to point to NAI.

A56 TFTFF
Inguinal herniae are almost always indirect in childhood and are more common in boys. The greater incidence on the right side is likely to be linked to the fact that the right testis descends after the left and the processus vaginalis is likely to remain patent on that side for longer. A brightly transilluminating swelling in an infant is most likely to be a hydrocoele, which will have disappeared by the age of 1 year in the majority of cases. Torsion of

an appendage, such as the hydatid of Morgagni, is a common cause of the 'acute scrotum' and may require surgical exploration if testicular torsion cannot be excluded clinically. Idiopathic scrotal oedema produces mild discomfort, together with redness and swelling that may extend beyond the scrotum, but the epididymis and testis are not involved. Mumps orchitis is an extremely rare complication in childhood and does not involve the epididymis.

A57 TFTTT
The arithmetic mean of n values, usually known simply as the mean or average, is the sum of *n* observations divided by *n*. The geometric mean is the *n*th root of the product of *n* values, which equates to the antilogarithm of the arithmetic mean of the logarithmic values. It is always smaller than the arithmetic mean. The mode is the most commonly occurring value and therefore cannot exist if there is no variation in frequency between values. The median is the middle obsevation in a sequence of observations. Neither the mode nor median are amenable to mathematical operations as, unlike the mean, they are not algebraically defined. In an asymmetrical distribution the mean is weighted by outlying observations so, in such cases, the median is often favoured as a measure of central tendency.

A58 TTFTT
In the normal lung some of the bronchial arterial blood passes to the pulmonary veins after it has perfused the bronchi. Another source of shunt is the coronary venous blood that drains into the left ventricle of the heart. Pathological causes include cyanotic cardiac disease and obstructive lung disease. The hypoxaemia caused by shunt cannot be corrected by 100% oxygen because the shunted blood is never exposed to the high alveolar Po_2. However, there will be some rise in arterial Po_2 because of the additional oxygenation of blood that has passed through the ventilated alveoli. Shunt does not usually result in a raised CO_2 because any increase caused by the shunt will stimulate ventilation until levels are normal.

A59 FTTFT
Complement is a group of serum proteins present in an inactive form that can be activated in one of two cascades, the classical and alternative pathways. Both lead to the same physiological consequences, which are opsonization, lysis and cellular activation. The two pathways use different initiation processes to result

in the activation of C3 which is the common connection between them. Some of the complement deficiencies can result in an increased susceptibility to recurrent pyogenic infections, the most severe problems being associated with C3 deficiency. Deficiency of one of the later complement components, C5 to C9, leads to a specific increased risk of neisserial infections resulting in recurrent attacks of meningococcal infection and severe gonococcal disease. In acute nephritis and membranoproliferative glomerulonephritis, C3 is depressed. Deficiency of C1 esterase inhibitor leads to spontaneous episodes of angio-oedema and occurs as an autosomal dominant disorder. Most of the complement deficiency syndromes result in a predisposition to autoimmune disease, particularly systemic lupus erythematosus. Sarcoidosis is not associated with abnormalities of complement.

A60 TFTTF
Nerves of the parasympathetic system leave the central nervous system through the III, VII, IX and X cranial nerves and from the sacral outflow (predominantly the second and third sacral nerves). Effects on the eye involve contraction of the iris (miosis) and contraction of the ciliary muscle for near vision. Stimulation of the heart causes a reduction in heart rate and atrioventricular conduction velocity. Parasympathetic stimulation also causes bronchoconstriction, relaxation of arterioles, increased gut motility and secretions, relaxation of gut sphincters and contraction of the gallbladder. The detrusor muscle of the urinary bladder contracts and the trigone and sphincter relax.

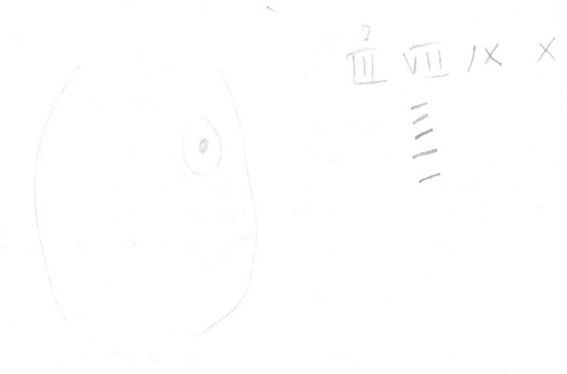

Practice examination B   Answers

B1 FFFTT
Damage to the ulnar nerve at the elbow leads to inability to adduct the thumb, spread the fingers, flex the metacarpophalangeal joints, or extend the interphalangeal joints, particularly of the ring and little fingers. This leads to the appearance of claw hand. Wrist drop results from damage to the radial nerve in the radial groove and opposition of the thumb and forefinger is supplied by the median nerve.

B2 TTFTT
Causes of neonatal hypoglycaemia can be classified as transient or persistent. Transient causes include intrauterine growth retardation, prematurity, birth asphyxia, sepsis, maternal diabetes, erythroblastosis fetalis, Beckwith–Wiedemann syndrome (may also be persistent), and maternal drugs (e.g. β-sympathomimetics and chlorpropamide). Persistent hypoglycaemia may be due to an inborn error of metabolism including glycogen storage disorder types I, II and IV, maple syrup urine disease, nesidioblastosis, galactosaemia and mitochondrial fatty acid oxidation defects such as MCAD deficiency. Hormonal deficiencies such as congenital hypopituitarism, congenital glucagon deficiency and cortisol deficiency states including congenital adrenal hypoplasia are also causes of persistent hypoglycaemia.

B3 FTTFF
Metabolic acidosis occurs from excessive accumulation of any acid in the body other than carbon dioxide. It occurs if the kidneys fail to excrete a normal acid load, in severe diarrhoea with loss of bicarbonate, in various inborn errors of metabolism or if there is anaerobic production of lactic acid from any other cause. The biochemical features are a high hydrogen ion concentration, low pH, low bicarbonate and a negative base excess. Plasma proteins have a reduced affinity for calcium in an acid environment and therefore ionized calcium levels rise. Acetazolamide is a carbonic anhydrase inhibitor which prevents adequate reabsorption of bicarbonate by the proximal renal tubules, thus leading to acidosis.

B4 TFFTT
Septal hypertrophy is one of the manifestations of macrosomia seen with hyperinsulinism in neonates and is usually self-limiting. Hypertrophic obstructive cardiomyopathy (HOCM) accounts for most cases in other age groups. It is mainly a disease of children, adolescents and young adults, is passed on by a mendelian dominant form of inheritance with incomplete penetrance. It is a

progressive condition and sudden death is a well recognized risk; 25% have mitral regurgitation. Beta-blockers are the mainstay of treatment, relieving symptoms of chest pain and breathlessness and allowing regression of the hypertrophy if started early. Verapamil, nifedipine or amiodarone may also be used, but only the latter has any influence on the incidence of sudden death. Friedreich's ataxia is associated with a similar cardiomyopathy which may precede the clinical onset of ataxia.

B5 FTFTF
Infective endocarditis is usually associated with an underlying cardiac lesion or intracardiac prosthesis, but children with structurally normal hearts can be affected. It is rare in infants and young children and much more common in adults. *Streptococcus viridans* and *Staphylococcus aureus* are the main causes of infection. Other bacteria or fungi may be isolated and in about 10% of cases no organism is identified from blood cultures. Patients at risk of developing infective endocarditis must have prophylactic antibiotic treatment for any procedure that may cause bacteraemia. However, these measures may be ineffective in up to 50% of cases. Complications of infective endocarditis include haematuria, valve damage, cerebral emboli, splinter haemorrhages and mild splenomegaly.

B6 TTTFF
Hypercyanotic attacks or spells are thought to occur because of spasm of the infundibular muscle, preventing pulmonary flow and increasing the right to left shunt across the ventricular septal defect. These life-threatening episodes commonly occur in infants who are normally pink and are often initiated by crying or exertion. During the attack the infant should be placed in the knee-elbow position to increase systemic vascular resistance and increase pulmonary blood flow. Oxygen at a concentration of 100% should be administered by a face mask. Intravenous propranolol may reverse the infundibular spasm and, following the attack, should be continued in an oral form as a prophylactic measure while awaiting surgery.

B7 FTTFF
Pulmonary hypertension is present when the mean pulmonary artery pressure is greater than 20 mmHg. Cardiac causes are due to increased pulmonary blood flow or pulmonary venous obstruction. Pulmonary atresia and Fallot's tetralogy lead to reduced pulmonary blood flow. Hypoxia due to chronic lung disease,

chronic upper airway obstruction (e.g. severe tonsillar hypertrophy) or non-respiratory causes such as high altitude or neurological hypoventilation can all lead to pulmonary hypertension. Diseases of the pulmonary vascular tree itself (primary pulmonary hypertension and thromboembolism) are also causes. There is no specific long-term treatment for pulmonary hypertension and identification of the cause with appropriate treatment is therefore essential.

B8 TTTTT
Erythema multiforme is a common skin condition, thought to be associated with immune complex deposition, leading to a widespread erythematous rash with macular, papular and vesicular components and characteristic target lesions, particularly on the extensor surfaces of the arms and legs. It is particularly associated with administration of sulphonamide or non-steroidal anti-inflammatory drugs and following infection with the herpes simplex virus or mycoplasma. Other infections which may be implicated are the Epstein Barr virus, causing infectious mononucleosis, orf, typhoid, diphtheria and focal bacterial sepsis, chlamydia and deep fungal infection with histoplasmosis. Radiotherapy, leukaemia and collagen diseases, such as systemic lupus erythematosus and polyarteritis nodosa, have also been described as causes.

B9 TFTTF
The Moro reflex and the asymmetrical tonic neck reflex, which results in increased extensor tone on the side to which the head is turned, and flexor tone on the other, are present from around 28 weeks' gestation and are abnormal if persistent beyond 6 months of age. The rooting, sucking, swallowing reflexes and the glabellar tap also appear around 28 weeks' gestation, whereas the stepping reflex appears a few weeks later and disappears by 2–3 months. The downward and forward parachute responses appear around 6 and 9 months respectively, and serve to protect the infant as he learns to move. The plantar or Babinski reflex is extensor (upgoing) in normal infants and is therefore not a useful test in the newborn.

B10 FTTFT
A 3 year old should be able to stand momentarily on one foot, but hopping starts on the favoured foot around age four. He should also be able to walk upstairs one foot per step and pedal a tricycle. Two year olds can kick a ball. Knowledge of full name,

sex, age and particularly address is very much dependent on environment, but most 3 year olds can give full name, age and sex, and failure by four indicates delay. Most 3 year olds have mastered eating with a spoon and fork, but use of knife and fork usually takes till beyond age four to develop.

B11 TFTFF
The endodermal germ layer develops into the lining of the gut, bladder and respiratory tract, including the eustachian tube, and the parenchyma of the tonsil, thyroid, parathyroids, thymus, liver and pancreas. The mesodermal germ layer gives rise to supporting tissues of the body, the vascular system, including spleen, the urogenital system, except bladder, and the adrenal cortex. Ectodermal structures are those which maintain contact with the outside world and include the central and peripheral nervous systems, including the adrenal medulla, sensory epithelia, the pituitary, mammary and sweat glands, the skin, hair, nails and enamel of the teeth.

B12 FTFTT
There are five phases of iron poisoning. In the first 2 h, as serum levels rise, acute cerebral and gastrointestinal effects may be seen, leading to massive blood and fluid loss with circulatory failure in the most severe cases. Serum levels then fall as hepatic deposition takes effect, and the symptoms may be quiescent for up to 48 h. Metabolic acidosis and peripheral circulatory failure may follow with increased capillary permeability adding to the problems of fluid loss. The fourth stage is hepatic necrosis after several days and the fifth, gastric or pyloric scarring causing obstruction some weeks after ingestion. Treatment includes gastric lavage which may need repeating if an abdominal X-ray demonstrates residual iron in the stomach. General supportive measures must be implemented and, at least in severe cases, administration of the chelating agent desferrioxamine, given intravenously. Oral instillation of desferrioxamine is of uncertain value and is not employed universally.

B13 FTTFT
More than 90% of cases of congenital adrenal hyperplasia are the result of 21 α-hydroxylase deficiency. Females are virilized and therefore present early with ambiguous genitalia. Males present with salt losing crises, which occur after the first few days of life. All varieties of congenital adrenal hyperplasia show autosomal recessive inheritance. Patients are sodium depleted so need

sodium chloride supplementation in addition to hydrocortisone and fludrocortisone. Fluid restriction would be dangerous. In 21 α-hydroxylase deficiency, amniotic fluid levels of 17-hydroxy-progesterone are grossly elevated in salt losers. The gene is closely linked to the HLA loci so, if the HLA type is known for both parents and the affected child, the fetal HLA type can be used for diagnosis. A gene probe is also available. All at risk pregnancies are covered with dexamethasone until the diagnosis is made, and continued only in the case of affected females.

B14 FFTTF
Somatomedin C was the name originally given to the hormone, now known as IGF-1, which exerted metabolic effects *in vitro*, closely resembling those of insulin. It is a polypeptide with 43% sequence homology with human pro-insulin. Synthesis occurs mainly in the liver but other tissues contribute to a lesser extent. Although IGF-1 is less potent than insulin in inducing hypogly-caemia, its effects are measurable. Its precise role in glucose homeostasis is unclear.

B15 FTTFT
Delayed bone age may occur in familial maturation delay, where a normal final height is attained without intervention but, in familial short stature, the bone age is normal. Bone age may be delayed in any systemic disorder, nutritional and emotional deprivation, and in a number of endocrine disorders; growth hormone deficiency may result from radiotherapy or an intracranial mass such as a craniopharyngioma. Hyperthyroidism leads to tall stature and advanced bone age, whereas Klinefelter syndrome, though associated with tall stature, usually results in delayed puberty and thus also delayed bone age.

B16 FTFTF
The anterior pituitary secretes the following hormones: adreno-corticotrophic hormone (ACTH), follicle stimulating hormone (FSH), luteinizing hormone (LH), melanocyte stimulating hormone (MSH), somatotrophin or growth hormone, thyroid stimulating hormone (TSH) and prolactin. Oxytocin and antidiuretic hormone are secreted by the posterior lobe of the pituitary.

B17 TFTTT
Conjugated hyperbilirubinaemia is a feature of disorders which cause intra- or extrahepatic obstruction to the excretion of bile. Inherited syndromes include Rotor syndrome, in which there is

impairment of the uptake and storage of bile, and Dubin–Johnson syndrome, where the defect is in bilirubin excretion. Cirrhosis from any cause, including haemochromatosis, causes obstructive jaundice. Viral hepatitis leads to raised levels of both conjugated and unconjugated bilirubin. Paroxysmal nocturnal haemoglobin-uria causes haemolysis due to a rare acquired red cell defect and the urine may be dark due to the presence of haemoglobin. As in other types of haemolysis, the additional circulating bilirubin is unconjugated, resulting from the failure of the conjugation process to keep up with the breakdown of haemoglobin. Conjugated bilirubin is water soluble and therefore passes across glomeruli into the urine, whereas unconjugated bilirubin circulates bound to albumin and is not filtered by normal glomeruli.

B18 FFTTF
In this age group the commonest causes of blood in the stool with abdominal pain are constipation and infection, in particular with *Campylobacter* and *Salmonella*. Other causes include gastritis, peptic ulcer, volvulus, Meckel's diverticulitis, mesenteric thrombosis, ulcerative colitis, ileitis and child abuse. Gastrointestinal involvement is fairly common in Henoch–Schönlein purpura (HSP) with bleeding into the gut wall causing colicky pain and fresh blood or melaena. Intussusception can also occur in HSP and needs to be excluded. Necrotizing enterocolitis is a disease of the neonate.

B19 FTFTT
Intussusception has a peak incidence at 6–9 months but can occur at any age. It classically presents with spasmodic pain and blood-stained mucous stools, and sometimes vomiting. A sausage-shaped mass may be palpable over the ascending or transverse colon. If there is a delay in diagnosis there may be signs of peritonitis. Laparotomy only identifies an underlying abnormality such as Meckel's diverticulum, lymphoma or polyp in 5% of cases, but this increases in older children. Management consists of resuscitation followed by reduction by barium or air enema. If radiological reduction fails or if there is evidence of peritonitis, operative reduction is indicated.

B20 FTTFT
Tuberous sclerosis is one of the neurodermatoses, conditions in which skin lesions are associated with neurological lesions and increased risk of tumour formation. There are four main dermatological manifestations. 'Adenoma sebaceum' is a misnomer

since these facial lesions are angiofibromata and therefore neither adenomata nor related to sebaceous glands. Periungual fibromata, appearing as fleshy papules under and around nails, occur around puberty and shagreen patches, irregularly thickened plaques usually seen over the lumbosacral area, appear in early childhood. Ash leaf depigmented macules, usually oval in shape, appear in infancy. Characteristic neurological features include infantile spasms, generalized epilepsy and mental retardation, although the latter is a particularly variable feature. Imaging of the brain may reveal multiple nodules or periventricular calcification. Other systemic manifestations include rhabdomyomata of the heart, which may lead to cyanotic attacks, retinal phakomata, renal tumours and cyst formation, cystic lesions of the lungs and occasional haemangiomata of the liver and spleen. Bone involvement is rare and polyostotic fibrous dysplasia of bone is seen as areas of rarefaction in patients with McCune–Albright syndrome (hyperpigmented macules, precocious puberty and bone changes). Tuberous sclerosis is inherited as an autosomal dominant character and two sites of mutation have been identified as deletions on the short arms of chromosomes 9 and 16.

B21 TTFFF
X-linked recessive traits result from a mutant gene on the X chromosome, carried by heterozygous females who are usually asymptomatic, and expressed in males who are hemizygous. (A hemizygous gene is one that is present in a single dose.) Both haemophilia A and B are inherited in this way. Other important X-linked disorders include G-6PD deficiency, chronic granulomatous disease, Lesch–Nyhan and Lowe's syndromes, Duchenne and Becker muscular dystrophies and Hunter's syndrome. Vitamin D dependent rickets, resulting either from a defect in the 1α-hydroxylase enzyme (type I) or end organ resistance (type II), is transmitted as an autosomal recessive trait. Hurler's syndrome is an autosomal recessive condition and Holt Oram autosomal dominant.

B22 FTTFT
The cell cycle consists of the M phase for mitosis, S phase during which DNA is replicated and the G or gap phases in between. G1, whose length varies most according to the rapidity with which a given cell type divides, precedes S, and G_2 follows. Differentiated cells, which are no longer dividing, are in the resting or G_0 phase, having left the cycle prior to S. The relationships between these phases are best appreciated in diagrammatic form, beyond the

scope of this book. Mitosis (nuclear division) is divided into five stages and is followed by cytokinesis (cytoplasmic division). Prophase marks the end of interphase and G_2 with condensation of the chromatin and formation of the spindle apparatus. This develops further during prometaphase, when the nuclear envelope breaks down. The chromosomes line up midway between the poles during metaphase, where the process is arrested in the presence of colchicine, and the sister chromatids are pulled to opposite poles in anaphase. Two nuclear envelopes form round the sets of chromosomes during telophase.

B23 TTFTT

Hypochromia, along with microcytosis, results from a defect in haemoglobin synthesis. The most common cause is iron deficiency. Malabsorption in coeliac disease may also lead to folate deficiency and produce a dimorphic picture. Hiatus hernia produces iron deficiency through chronic blood loss. All of the thalassaemias may give a microcytic hypochromic appearance to the blood film although the thalassaemia traits may not produce anaemia. The anaemia of chronic disease generally leads to a normochromic normocytic picture but hypochromia is also frequently seen. Other causes of hypochromia include lead poisoning and sideroblastic anaemia. Sickle cell disease gives rise to a haemolytic anaemia with sickle cells, target cells and Howell–Jolly bodies seen on the blood film.

B24 TTFTT

In haemophilia A (classical haemophilia) there is a prolonged partial thromboplastin time, with a normal prothrombin time and fibrinogen. The prothrombin time is a measure of the extrinsic coagulation pathway and the partial thromboplastin time measures the intrinsic pathway. Factor IX is low in haemophilia B (Christmas disease), but is normal in haemophilia A.

B25 FTTFF

Transfusion associated graft versus host disease (TA-GvHD) may follow transfusion of blood products containing viable T cells. Irradiation destroys these cells. TA-GvHD usually occurs in children with congenital abnormalities of cell-mediated immunity like DiGeorge syndrome or during treatment for malignancy. It has not been reported in acquired T cell deficiency such as HIV infection. For children receiving standard chemotherapy the risk is very low and irradiation of blood products is therefore not recommended. However, those undergoing bone marrow transplant are considered at higher risk and should therefore receive irradiated products.

B26 FFTTT

Kawasaki disease is of unknown aetiology. It is most common in girls between 2 months and 9 years of age and usually presents with a persistent fever. It is diagnosed on clinical grounds when five of the following six features are present: fever for more than 5 days; polymorphous exanthematous rash; cervical lymphadenopathy; non-purulent conjunctivitis; oral mucosal changes; and erythema oedema or desquamation of hands and feet. Fewer criteria are accepted if there is echocardiographic or post-mortem evidence of coronary artery abnormalities. No diagnostic test is available but laboratory findings include a high ESR, high CRP, leucocytosis, thrombocytosis and raised $\alpha2$ globulin. Untreated, 15–40% develop coronary artery aneurysms. Other complications include pericarditis and myocarditis, arthritis, aseptic meningitis, pancreatitis and hydrops of the gallbladder.

B27 TFFTF

Neonates are immunocompromised, particularly if premature. The newborn is deficient in IgA and IgM. IgG is actively transported across the placenta from 32 weeks' gestation resulting in a level equal to or more than that of an adult. However, some subclasses are not transferred resulting in deficiency. Complement levels are only 50% of adult levels, and although there are adequate numbers of B cells their immunoglobulin production is reduced. T cell function may be reduced and there is inadequate T and B cell interaction.

B28 TFTTT

Secondary immunodeficiency is more common than primary immunodeficiency. It may follow radiotherapy and treatment with drugs including cytotoxics, corticosteroids, phenytoin and cyclosporin A. Nephrotic syndrome and burns lead to immunoglobulin deficiency through protein loss and in myotonic dystrophy there is increased catabolism of immunoglobulin. Many viral infections can lead to lymphopenia and abnormal white cell response to infection. A child with congenital rubella or cytomegalovirus infection may have markedly reduced antibody responses and hypogammaglobulinaemia. Septicaemia or infections with protozoa (e.g. malaria) also adversely affect immune function. Hyposplenism, which may result from sickle cell disease, results in an increased risk of infection with pneumococcus and other polysaccharide encapsulated organisms. Other important causes of secondary immunodeficiency include malignancy and malnutrition. Haematological complications associated with sodium valproate are thrombocytopenia and failure of platelet aggregation but there are no effects on immunity.

B29 TTTFT
Both primary and congenital infection with toxoplasmosis may be asymptomatic. Symptomatic acquired infection may be limited to cervical lymphadenopathy or may mimic infectious mononucleosis. More complicated cases may develop chorioretinitis (rare in the acquired form), hepatitis, myocarditis, encephalitis, myositis and arthritis. Clinical features of the congenital infection include hydrocephaly, chorioretinitis and intracranial calcification most commonly, but microphthalmia, cataract, deafness, hepatosplenomegaly, lymphadenopathy, pneumonitis, cardiac lesions and intrauterine growth retardation are also well recognized. Recurrence in infants of subsequent pregnancies is rare but is thought to result from the persistence of the organism as cysts in the myometrium. Toxoplasmosis is associated with lymphocytosis.

B30 TTFFT
Statutorily notifiable diseases, under the Public Health (Control of Diseases) Act 1984 and the Public Health (Infectious Diseases) Regulations 1988, are:

Acute encephalitis	Measles	Scarlet fever
Acute poliomyelitis	Meningitis	Smallpox
Anthrax	Meningococcal sepsis	Tetanus
Cholera	Mumps	Tuberculosis
Diphtheria	Ophthalmia neonatorum	Typhoid fever
Dysentery	Paratyphoid fever	Typhus
Food poisoning	Plague	Viral haemorrhagic fever
Leprosy	Rabies	Viral hepatitis
Leptospirosis	Relapsing fever	Whooping cough
Malaria	Rubella	Yellow fever

B31 TTTFF
The incubation periods for the infections listed are as follows: chicken pox, 14–21 days; pertussis, 7–14 days; herpes simplex

viruses, 3–14 days; measles, 8–14 days and coxsackie viruses, between 2 and 9 days.

B32 TTTTF
Adenovirus infection most commonly causes upper respiratory tract infections but there are numerous subtypes and the spectrum of clinical disease is very wide, including lower respiratory infections, gastroenteritis, conjunctivitis and haemorrhagic cystitis. Disseminated infection, leading to involvement of the CNS, heart or liver, is occasionally seen but more likely in the immunocompromised. Slapped cheek disease, or erythema infectiosum, is caused by parvovirus infection.

B33 TFFFT
Still's disease, or systemic onset juvenile chronic arthritis, typically presents in children under the age of 5 years. There may be no joint involvement at presentation, symptoms being high spiking fever, rash, lymphadenopathy and splenomegaly. White blood cell and platelet counts may be raised, and a high ESR is expected, but rheumatoid factor and antinuclear antibodies are rarely found. Iridocyclitis is unusual, being more characteristic of the pauciarticular variety, particularly in the presence of antinuclear antibody. Still's murmur, a buzzing or vibratory murmur heard maximally at the lower left sternal edge, is an unrelated finding.

B34 TTFFT
NEC is a condition of combined infection and ischaemia of the bowel wall, and is most commonly seen in preterm neonates. Precise aetiology is unclear but it is associated with perinatal asphyxia, particularly when reversed end-diastolic flow in the umbilical artery has been demonstrated *in utero* in the growth retarded infant. Other predisposing factors include respiratory distress, prolonged antepartum rupture of membranes, sepsis, jaundice, twin delivery, caesarean section, congenital heart disease, hyperosmolar feeds and abnormalities of the bowel, such as Hirschsprung's disease. The early introduction of feeds in at risk infants may contribute to NEC and breast milk may be protective, compared to artificial formulae.

B35 TTTTT
Hydrops fetalis, universal oedema of the fetus, may be the end point of a large number of conditions and has many associations. The mechanisms are disputed but severe anaemia, congestive

cardiac failure and hypoproteinaemia all play a part. Aetiologies include haematological, cardiovascular, pulmonary, renal, gastrointestinal, hepatic, neoplastic and infective disorders, chromosomal and other congenital anomalies, placental conditions, maternal diabetes, toxaemia and anaemia. About half of the cases of non-immunological hydrops are idiopathic.

B36 FTFTT
New nephrons only continue to form until the 36th week of gestation. Thereafter there is an increase in the tubular length and glomerular size. The glomerular filtration rate, renal bicarbonate reabsorption and glucose reabsorption are all markedly reduced in comparison to adult values when corrected for size. The urea excretion is greatly reduced, and normal blood urea levels are due to relatively more dietary nitrogen deposited as protein in the tissue, and anabolism and growth.

B37 FFFTF
Surfactant deficient respiratory distress syndrome (RDS) is caused by surfactant deficiency and is usually associated with prematurity. Other factors that increase the incidence include maternal diabetes, antepartum haemorrhage, birth asphyxia, twin pregnancy, male sex and previous family history. Factors that are associated with a decreased incidence are intrauterine growth retardation, maternal steroid therapy, sickle cell disease, female sex and infants of Afrocaribbean origin.

B38 TTFFF
Hypoalbuminaemia in minimal change nephrotic syndrome leads to varying degrees of intravascular volume depletion. The resulting outpouring of antidiuretic hormone (ADH) may contribute to a drop in plasma sodium which is frequently found to be low in the acute phase. Daily urine estimations of protein, using dipsticks, are the mainstay of monitoring and can be used to guide treatment. Serum albumin estimations, although frequently made, add very little information, once the diagnosis is made, except in the most severe cases. Only the most severe cases require albumin infusions; poor perfusion and severe oedema, particularly of the external genitalia, resulting from severe hypoalbuminaemia, being the main indications. Frusemide is usually given in conjunction with albumin, to prevent pulmonary oedema resulting from sudden large fluid shifts. Disease control is generally achieved with oral corticosteroids but 70% relapse after the first course.

B39 FFFTT

A substance for measuring glomerular filtration rate (GFR) should not be protein bound, metabolized, secreted or absorbed by the tubules and should be freely filtered. Inulin is suitable as it meets these criteria but measurement using the radioisotope ^{51}Cr-EDTA is often preferred as its clearance may be measured without the need for urine colleciton. Creatinine is often used for clinical estimation of the GFR but its use is limited as it is sometimes absorbed or secreted by the tubules. GFR is maintained when efferent arteriolar resistance to blood flow is greater than afferent. Sympathetic stimulation preferentially constricts the afferent renal arterioles, decreasing pressure in the glomerular capillaries and therefore reducing the GFR. Cisplatin treatment leads to both glomerular and renal tubular damage.

B40 FFFTT

All recorded cases of Rett syndrome are female. Familial recurrence is documented but rare. Most cases are thought to be new mutations, although X-linked dominant transmission has been suggested. Initial developmental progress, up to at least 6 months and sometimes up to 18 months, is usually normal. After this time, regression occurs, and previously learned skills are gradually lost. The hands are often the key to diagnosis, with the development of abnormal movements, including hand clasping, wringing and washing actions.

B41 TTFFF

Absence seizures usually start between 3 and 10 years of age with a peak at 6 years. The seizures typically last 5–20 s. The child suddenly becomes still and the eyes stare or drift upwards. There may be flickering of the eyelids. At the end of the episode the child continues with the activity he was involved with. Initial treatment is with ethosuximide or sodium valproate. Absences rarely persist into adolescence, but up to 40% of patients will go on to develop tonic–clonic seizures at some stage.

B42 TTFFT

Subacute sclerosing panencephalitis (SSPE) usually complicates measles infection some 5–10 years after initial infection. It appears more frequently if primary measles occurs under the age of 1 year. Early signs are gradual deterioration of intellectual performance and behavioural problems. This is followed by involuntary movements, spasticity, visual disturbance, nystagmus and optic atrophy. Extrapyramidal signs and seizures occur in the later stages. The electroencephalogram characteristically shows burst suppression. There are high titres of measles antibody in both the serum and the cerebrospinal fluid (CSF). The CSF has normal or mildly raised protein and the cells are either normal or there are increased mononuclear cells. The incidence of SSPE has fallen since the introduction of measles vaccination.

B43 FTTFT
Thiamine is a cofactor of many enzyme reactions. Body stores are small, but it is found in many foodstuffs so that deficiency is only seen where the only food consumed is polished rice, and in chronic alcoholics who eat virtually no food. It presents with one of two types of beri-beri: (a) in wet beri-beri swelling occurs due to inadequate metabolism of glucose resulting in lactate and pyruvate accumulation producing peripheral vasodilation and oedema. Heart muscle may be affected resulting in failure. (b) In dry beri-beri there is a polyneuropathy and possible cerebral involvement (Wernicke–Korsakoff syndrome). The response to treatment with thiamine is dramatic in wet beri-beri but very slow in the dry form. Niacin deficiency results in pellagra.

B44 TTFTF
Maternal malnutrition reduces the volume and fat content of milk but has negligible effect on the protein content. Human milk contains less vitamin K than formula milk and cases of haemor-rhagic disease are described more frequently in breast fed babies. Breast fed babies have a lower stool pH favouring colonization by *Lactobacillus* and inhibiting growth of *E. coli*. Immunological properties of breast milk range from macrophages and non-specific immune factors to specific passive immunity conferred by secretory IgA and the stimulation of the infant's immune system by mechanisms which have not been fully elucidated.

B45 FTFFT
In childhood ALL a high initial leucocyte count is associated with a poor prognosis. Children with blast cells showing common ALL antigen achieve higher survival rates than those with T or B cell markers. Other poor prognostic factors include central nervous system involvement at diagnosis, age below 2 or above 10 years and male sex.

B46 TTFFF
If normal binocular use of the eyes is prevented, central suppression of one eye leads to development of amblyopia, or lazy eye. It is

classically the result of uncorrected non-paralytic squint or severe refractive error in childhood, but may also result from cataract, ptosis or corneal opacities. Childhood squint may also lead to abnormal head posture, sometimes mistaken for torticollis. Paralytic squint is more commonly an acquired disorder in older patients, following trauma, vascular accidents, aneurysms or tumours. The cover test is used to diagnose squint. The diagnosis of amblyopia relies on the demonstration of reduced acuity in one eye without a detectable disorder of the retina or visual pathways, so assessment should include detailed ophthalmoscopy. Amblyopia is likely to be irreversible if it persists beyond the age of 7 years, whereas it will usually resolve within weeks if the cause is treated in infancy.

B47 TTTFF
Bactericidal antibiotics include β-lactams (penicillin and cephalosporin groups), aminoglycosides, polymyxins, rifampicin, nalidixic acid and metronidazole. Fusidic acid and macrolides such as erythromycin may be bactericidal in high dosage, but are bacteristatic in low doses. Other bacteristatic antibiotics include sulphonamides, tetracyclines and trimethoprim.

B48 FFTFT
Alprostadil is indicated to maintain the patency of the ductus arteriosus temporarily until corrective or palliative surgery can be performed in infants who have congenital heart defects dependent on the ductus for perfusion of the pulmonary arteries. It should be administered by continuous intravenous infusion. Up to 10% of neonates treated with alprostadil experience apnoea. Other side effects include pyrexia, bradycardia, seizures, hypotension and gastric outflow obstruction secondary to antral hyperplasia. No drug interactions have been reported to occur with standard treatments used in neonates with congenital heart disease.

B49 TFFTF
1 kg = 1000 g
1 g = 1000 mg
1 mg = 1000 μg
1 μg = 1000 ng

Adrenaline 1:1000 = 1 mg/ml
Adrenaline 1:10 000 = 1 mg/10 ml

Lignocaine 2% = 20 mg/ml
Sodium bicarbonate 8.4% = 1 mmol/ml

Sodium chloride 0.9% = 150 mmol/l sodium
Glucose 4% + saline 0.18% = 31 mmol/l sodium
Human albumin solution 4.5% contains approximately 150 mmol/l sodium.

B50 TTFTT

The principal side effect of morphine is respiratory depression. It is also a potent antitussive and sometimes causes bronchospasm. It has minimal effects on the cardiovascular system, but may cause hypotension which is partially mediated by histamine release. In high doses it may cause a bradycardia. Morphine decreases gut motility and reduces gastric acid, biliary and pancreatic secretion. It causes spasm of the sphincter of Oddi and may lead to nausea, vomiting, and constipation. Morphine increases the secretion of antidiuretic hormone and may therefore lead to impaired water excretion and hyponatraemia.

B51 FFFTT

Anorexia nervosa is a condition which mainly affects adolescent females, with an increased incidence in middle and upper social classes. Males account for 5–10% of cases. It is characterized by self-induced weight loss to more than 15% below the expected percentile and refusal to maintain a reasonable body weight. The patient has a disturbed body image and an intense fear of becoming obese, believing she is fat, although aware that others regard her as thin. This is an overvalued idea rather than a delusion as it does not have the quality of unshakeable conviction. The condition starts with a gradual reduction in the intake of food which is eventually extended to fluids. Strategies such as excessive exercise, vomiting and the abuse of laxatives and diuretics are employed to increase weight loss. Consequences of starvation include poor circulation with bradycardia, hypotension, low body temperature and impaired peripheral perfusion, amenorrhoea, which occasionally precedes weight loss, and the development of 'lanugo' hair.

B52 FTFTT

Questions on the oxyhaemoglobin dissociation curve are popular with examiners but the wording may be confusing. Sketching the curve may help answering this sort of question, particularly when under stress. A rightward shift of the curve corresponds to increased unloading of oxygen at a given Po_2 in the capillaries. A shift to the right is caused by an increase in hydrogen ion concentration, Pco_2, temperature and the concentration of diphosphoglycerate (2,3 DPG). An exercising muscle is acidic, hypercarbic and hot, and it benefits from increased unloading of oxygen from the capillaries. A useful measure of the position of the curve is the P50 which is the Po_2 for 50% oxygen saturation. Adult Hb has a lower affinity for oxygen than fetal Hb to assist oxygen transfer across the placenta. HbS results in a shift of the curve to the right in addition to the cell shape changes and increased cell fragility.

B53 FTFFF
Hyperventilation causes respiratory alkalosis by removing sufficient carbon dioxide from the body to reduce hydrogen ion concentration and increase the pH. With time the kidneys compensate for this loss of CO_2 by secreting bicarbonate. Plasma proteins have an increased affinity for calcium in an alkaline environment. The resultant hypocalcaemia leads to increased excitability of the central and peripheral nervous systems with tetany and seizures. Vasodilation of cerebral vessels occurs in response to hypoventilation and hypercapnia.

B54 TTFFT
Pneumococcus is the most common cause of childhood pneumonia. Cytomegalovirus pneumonia usually only affects children with immunodeficiency. The symptoms associated with pneumonia caused by *Mycoplasma pneumoniae* are often much worse than the physical signs would suggest. Staphylococcal pneumonia is a rare disease in healthy children and should alert the clinician to the possibility of cystic fibrosis. *Pneumocystis carinii* pneumonia is an opportunistic infection seen in the immunocompromised and may be treated with co-trimoxazole.

B55 FTTFT
Parental responsibility is automatic for the mother but for the father only if the parents are married. If they are unmarried, the father is awarded joint responsibility only on the basis of the mother's consent. Police may take a child into police protection if there are reasonable grounds for believing that the child may otherwise suffer significant harm. An emergency Protection Order may then be applied for if required, which stands for 8 days. Parental responsibility is not transferred under assessment orders or under police protection. Under the terms of the act, considerable emphasis is placed on the rights of the child.

B56 FTFFT
Sensitivity = true positives/(true positives + false negatives)
Specificity = true negatives/(true negatives + false positives)

Predictive value = true positives/(true positives + false positives)

False positives in a screening test will be eliminated by further investigation, whereas false negatives will not be detected so it is more important to design a test where the latter are minimized. The Guthrie test provides a good example of such a test, as it leads to very few false negatives, despite a large number of false positives, which are eliminated by further testing. It is a good example of an ideal screening test in other respects as it is a cheap test involving minimal discomfort, phenylketonuria is common enough to justify mass screening and is amenable to presymptomatic treatment. In cystic fibrosis there is controversy as to whether early treatment, with prophylactic antibiotics and physiotherapy, affects outcome. Screening is therefore not universally available. In centres where it is routine, it may lead to early intervention and also alerts families to the need for antenatal diagnosis in subsequent pregnancies, in cases where the index case may not otherwise have been diagnosed in time.

B57 FTFFF

The correlation coefficient between a random sample of values of two variables x and y is usually given as r and relates to the interdependence between the variables. Its magnitude indicates the strength of the linear relationship between x and y but has no implications on cause or effect. If $r = 0$, there is no linear relationship whereas, if $r = +1$, there is perfect correlation and y increases with x, with all values on a straight line. If $r = -1$, there is also perfect correlation but y decreases as x increases. In regression, an equation is determined to express the dependence of one variable on another and used to produce a line of best fit between the two variables. Correlation is mathematically related to regression but r does not represent the gradient of the regression line.

B58 FTFTT

Carbon dioxide (CO_2) is transported in the blood to the lungs as dissolved CO_2 (7%), bicarbonate ions (70%) and carbaminohaemoglobin (23%). The Haldane effect describes the displacement of CO_2 from the blood when oxygen (O_2) binds to haemoglobin, as occurs in the alveolar capillaries. This displacement occurs because haemoglobin is a stronger acid when bound to O_2 and has less affinity for CO_2 when acidic. Approximately 70% of CO_2 enters erythrocytes where it reacts with water to form carbonic acid under the influence of carbonic anhydrase. The carbonic acid dissociates into hydrogen ions and bicarbonate. The hydrogen ions combine with haemoglobin and the bicarbonate diffuses out of the cell. Henry's Law expresses the amount of gas that can be dissolved in a given volume of fluid.

B59 TFTFF

The bacteria most frequently isolated in neonatal meningitis are *E. coli* and group B streptococcus. *Listeria monocytogenes* is an important but rarer cause. *H. influenzae* used to be a common pathogen during early infancy, but it is now rare since the introduction of *H. influenzae* B into the vaccination schedule. Meningococcal disease tends to occur in older infants and children, although it may affect patients of any age. *Staph. aureus* and *Staph. epidermidis* are unlikely unless a ventricular shunt is *in situ*.

B60 TFTFT

Catecholamines acting at β_2 receptors cause vasodilatation, bronchoconstriction, relaxation of the smooth muscle of the gastrointestinal tract, relaxation of the uterine wall and detrusor muscle of the bladder, glycogenolysis and lipolysis.

Practice examination C   Answers

C1 TTFFT

Upper motor neuron lesions result from damage to the central nervous system, including the spinal cord, and result in weakness of voluntary movements and increased tone in affected muscles. The latter effect is a consequence of persistence of the stretch reflex which is normally suppressed by the descending tracts. Pain and temperature sensations are transmitted by the spinothalamic system whose tracts run in the contralateral white matter of the spinal cord. Discriminative touch, vibration sense and proprioception are transmitted by the dorsal columns which ascend ipsilaterally in the spinal cord and cross the midline in the caudal half of the medulla oblongata. The superficial reflexes, including the abdominal reflex and cremasteric reflex, are suppressed or absent in upper motor neuron lesions, in contrast to tendon jerks, which are exaggerated.

C2 FTTTF

Galactosaemia has an incidence of 1 in 60 000 and autosomal recessive inheritance. It is caused by deficiency of galactose-1-phosphate (gal-1-P) uridyl transferase and toxic effects result from accumulation of gal-1-P in the liver, kidney, lens and brain. It usually presents soon after the introduction of lactose in milk feeds and features include vomiting, jaundice, acidosis, hypoglycaemia, hepatomegaly, cataracts, failure to thrive and developmental delay. The clinical picture is easily confused with septicaemia and may also be complicated by septic episodes, particularly with *E.coli* in the newborn period. Cataracts may be present at birth, indicating that endogenous production of gal-1-P may occur *in utero*, although a milder subclinical enzyme deficiency in the heterozygous mother is also likely to contribute. Although screening for galactosaemia is carried out in some centres, most cases present early with symptoms before the results of screening would be available.

C3 FFTFF

The main circulating form of vitamin D is 25-hydroxycholecalciferol, formed in the liver from cholecalciferol. It is then hydroxylated further in the kidney to 24,25-dihydroxycholecalciferol and to its active form 1,25-dihydroxycholecalciferol. This causes increased calcium absorption and reabsorption in the intestine and renal tubules respectively and works together with parathyroid hormone to release calcium from bone. Deficiency of vitamin D leads to lowered plasma phosphate, together with calcium, whereas hypoparathyroidism causes hyperphosphataemia and hypocalcaemia.

C4 FTTFF

Four types of innocent murmur are recognized: a short systolic murmur with a musical or vibratory quality, heard along the left sternal edge; a soft systolic murmur in the pulmonary area; a short systolic murmur in the aortic area; and a continuous venous hum, heard over the base and in the neck. In general, innocent murmurs are short, systolic, localized, variable with respiration and posture, accentuated by fever and exercise, and not associated with a thrill, abnormalities of the heart sounds or signs of heart failure.

C5 FTTTF

Viral myocarditis is most commonly due to coxsackie B, but it may result from a variety of other viruses including mumps, cytomegalovirus (CMV) and adenovirus. It may rarely complicate a bacteraemia or infections with toxoplasma or candida. Diphtheria exotoxin may affect the conducting tissue with possible development of complete heart block. The course of viral myocarditis is variable, ranging from full recovery or chronic disability due to dilated cardiomyopathy to death. ECG changes are non-specific.

C6 TFFFT

During an episode of supraventricular tachycardia (SVT) the ECG shows a rate of 220–300 per minute. The prognosis for attacks occurring in infancy is generally very good, although in older children attacks can occur repetitively for years. With infants who are not acutely ill the diving reflex can be attempted to abort the attack. If this does not work intravenous adenosine may be administered. Adenosine acts by preventing passage of the electrical impulse through the AV node and may stop an episode when given by fast i.v. bolus. Other treatments commonly used to abort attacks include d.c. cardioversion and digoxin.

C7 TFFFF

The catheter data given suggest that this patient has a large ventricular septal defect with left to right shunting (high O_2 saturation in the right ventricle) and severe pulmonary hypertension (the pulmonary pressures are equal to the systemic blood pressure). If there was pulmonary stenosis, as in Fallot's tetralogy, the pulmonary vasculature would be protected against high blood flow and therefore against pulmonary hypertension, and the shunt across the defect might be right to left rather than left to right. This patient would not be suitable for corrective surgery if the pulmonary hypertension is not reversible. Further investigation is therefore necessary prior to operating to assess reduction of the pulmonary vascular resistance using a pulmonary vasodilator. Since the femoral artery oxygen saturation is 96%, the boy would not be cyanosed.

C8 TTTTF
Erythema multiforme usually fades spontaneously within 10 days and only the less common severe manifestations of Stevens–Johnson syndrome receive treatment with corticosteroids. The lesions of urticaria pigmentosa usually develop between 1 and 9 months of age and resolve over a period of years. Eosinophilic granuloma is the most benign form of Langerhan's cell histiocytosis (or histiocytosis X), which may produce yellowish brown papules on the skin. Eczema herpeticum, caused by secondary infection of atopic eczema with herpes simplex leading to the risk of further bacterial infection, usually requires treatment with systemic antibacterial and sometimes also antiviral therapy.

C9 TFTFT
Many 1 year olds are walking alone but the average is 13 or 14 months. Development of vocabulary is variable, and its interpretation by parents subjective at best, but few would have words with meaning other than 'Mama', 'Dada'. The development of object permanence, where the child continues to look for a toy after it is removed from sight, is a useful milestone and easy to test. A pincer grasp is developed around 10 months of age, but the ability to pick up very small items less than 1 mm in diameter is generally considered an 18 month milestone.

C10 FTFTF
Learning difficulties are only found in a few cases of Klinefelter syndrome. Of the mucopolysaccharidoses, Hurler's and Sanfilippo syndromes result in learning difficulties but not Morquio disease.

C11 TTFTF
The mesodermal germ layer gives rise to supporting tissues of the body, the vascular system, including spleen, the urogenital system, except bladder, and the adrenal cortex. Ectodermal structures are those which maintain contact with the outside world and include the central and peripheral nervous systems, including the adrenal medulla, sensory epithelia, the pituitary, mammary and sweat glands, the skin, hair, nails and enamel of the teeth. The endodermal germ layer develops into the lining of the gut, bladder and respiratory tract, including the eustachian tube, and the

parenchyma of the tonsil, thyroid, parathyroids, thymus, liver and pancreas.

C12 TTFTT

Theophylline toxicity may cause vomiting, haematemesis, agitation, pupillary dilatation, convulsions and coma. The characteristic metabolic disturbance is hypokalaemia, which may develop very rapidly and is associated with metabolic alkalosis. Hyperglycaemia is also recognized. Sinus tachycardia is common and ventricular arrhythmias may occur in severe cases. Treatment should include emptying the stomach, and elimination may be enhanced by the administration of activated charcoal. Convulsions can be treated with diazepam, and hypokalaemia with infusions of potassium chloride. Intravenous administration of propranolol may be of benefit in cases of severe tachycardia and may also help correct the hypokalaemia and hyperglycaemia, but this treatment should be used with caution given the likelihood of asthma in a child exposed to a source of theophyllines.

C13 TFTFF

Features of congenital hypothyroidism include unconjugated jaundice, dry mottled skin, umbilical hernia, hoarse cry, coarse facial features, periorbital oedema, large tongue, hypothermia, slow feeding, constipation, large anterior fontanelle and persistent posterior fontanelle (but not an extra third fontanelle, as seen in Down's syndrome). Mental retardation is likely if congenital hypothyroidism is not diagnosed by the age of 3 months, but has been almost completely eradicated by the practice of screening.

C14 TTFTF

Gonadotrophin releasing hormone (GnRH) secretion is active well before the onset of puberty. Although up to 3% of normal boys enter puberty by the age of 9, there is a relatively high incidence of intracranial pathology in males with central precocious puberty, compared with females. Premature thelarche (breast development only) is a benign condition which may be seen as early as 2 years and requires no treatment. Testicular volume less than 4 ml is prepubertal. The growth spurt accompanies pubertal stages 2–3 in girls (average age 12) but does not occur until stage 4 (average age 14) in boys.

C15 TFFTF

Growth hormone secretion is regulated by a number of physiological and pharmacological variables, including the secretion of releasing and inhibitory hormones by the hypothalamus as well as physiological and pharmacological circumstances. Secretion is also stimulated by stress, sleep, hypoglycaemia, fasting, dopaminergic agonists and oestrogens. Pregnancy, hyperglycaemia and cortisol inhibit the release of growth hormone.

C16 FFTTF
Insulin is an anabolic hormone facilitating the use of carbohydrates for energy while depressing the use of fats and amino acids. It promotes glucose uptake and storage in the liver and facilitates glucose uptake by skeletal muscles. The membranes of brain cells are not dependent on insulin for permeability to glucose. Insulin secretion from the β-cells of the pancreatic islets is mostly controlled via a negative feedback effect of the blood glucose concentration. It is stimulated by β-agonists, acetylcholine and glucagon and inhibited by β-antagonists, α-agonists, somatostatin and thiazide diuretics.

C17 TFTTT
Wilson's disease, or hepatolenticular degeneration, is caused by impaired biliary excretion of copper and reduced incorporation into caeruloplasmin. It usually presents with the gradual onset of liver disease in childhood. Other manifestations include encephalopathy, due to deposition of copper in the basal ganglia, proximal renal tubular dysfunction and haemolysis. Slit lamp examination of the eyes may reveal Kayser–Fleischer rings, seen as greenish brown corneal deposits. Serum levels of caeruloplasmin are low and of copper are low or normal. Urinary copper is raised and may be increased further by a penicillamine load.

C18 TFTTF
Most causes of chronic diarrhoea can lead to failure to thrive. Crohn's disease is rare in early childhood but does occur. Toddler diarrhoea is common in well, thriving young children with normal weight gain. Malabsorption, as seen with cystic fibrosis, Schwachmann's syndrome and coeliac disease, allergies and infection, particularly due to giardia, are all possible causes of failure to thrive and diarrhoea.

C19 TTTFT
Causes of prolonged unconjugated hyperbilirubinaemia include breast milk jaundice, hypothyroidism, intestinal stasis with increased enterohepatic circulation of bilirubin, haemolytic

disease, sepsis and congenital infections. Rotor syndrome tends to present later in childhood with conjugated hyperbilirubinaemia.

C20 TFTFT
Pancreatic juice contains enzymes to digest protein, carbohydrate and fats, and bicarbonate ions to neutralize the acid chyme from the stomach. The proteolytic enzymes are trypsin, chymotrypsin, carboxypolypeptidase, ribonuclease and deoxyribonuclease. Pancreatic amylase digests carbohydrates, and fats are digested by lipase and cholesterol esterase. The enzymes are secreted by the acini of the pancreatic glands and bicarbonate ions by the epithelial cells of the small ductules leading from the acini.

C21 TTFFF
Dubin–Johnson and ataxia telangiectasia are subject to autosomal recessive inheritance. Wiskott–Aldrich syndrome is an X-linked recessive condition and hereditary spherocytosis is autosomal dominant. Treacher–Collins syndrome is thought to be autosomal dominant with incomplete penetrance and variable expressivity.

C22 TTFFT
Anticipation is the phenomenon where successive generations are affected more severely or at an earlier age by an inherited condition. Fragile X syndrome, Huntingdon disease and myotonic dystrophy are all characterized by recurring series of three bases, known as triplet repeats. These tend to increase in number from one generation to the next and are related to the severity of the phenotype. Angelman syndrome is an example of imprinting, where the phenotype is dependent on the parental origin of the mutant gene(s) and Leber's optic atrophy is caused by a defect in mitochondrial DNA.

C23 FTFTF
The karyotype of Klinefelter syndrome is 47XXY with a low risk of recurrence and variable phenotype. Features include tall stature with long limbs, female fat distribution and gynaecomastia, small testes and normal or mildly impaired intellect. Presentation may be as delayed puberty or incomplete virilization, requiring testosterone treatment, or as infertility. Incidence of breast cancer is similar to that of normal females and an increased incidence of leukaemia is suggested by some sources.

C24 TFFTF
When haemoglobin is first synthesized *in utero*, HbA constitutes less than 10% of the total but rises to approximately 30% at term.

HbF falls to 10% by 4 months, but takes several years to reach adult levels of 1%. HbA$_2$, made up of α and δ globin polypeptide chains, constitutes 2.5% of normal haemoglobin from 4 months. In β thalassaemia, levels are much higher, to compensate for reduced levels or absence of β-chains, needed to make up HbA. Homozygous α thalassaemia results from deletion of all four α-globin genes, leading to Barts hydrops fetalis, with haemoglobin types Hb Barts (γ4), HbH (β4) and HB Portland. Beta thalassaemia can only be reliably diagnosed in late infancy, once HbF has fallen in normal subjects.

C25 TFTTF
The prothrombin time measures the extrinsic coagulation pathway. It is abnormal when oral anticoagulants are used, in liver disease, haemorrhagic disease of the newborn, DIC and vitamin K deficiency.

C26 FTTTF
Reticulocytes are immature red blood cells. Under normal conditions they remain in the marrow for about 24 h and are then released into the circulation, where they lose their RNA and become mature erythrocytes. Usually not more than 2% of peripheral red cells are reticulocytes, but their numbers are greatly increased if there is increased erythropoiesis, for example following blood loss or haemolysis. Aplastic anaemia (e.g. Fanconi's anaemia) results in pancytopenia associated with very few reticulocytes. Iron deficiency anaemia is associated with a low reticulocyte count but a reticulyte response may be sought once treatment is underway.

C27 TTFTF
Henoch–Schönlein or anaphylactoid purpura (HSP) is a systemic vasculitis of unknown aetiology, most commonly seen among preschool children. Renal involvement occurs in 25–50% of children and may occur up to 3 months after the rash. It is usually self-limiting but may progress to irreversible renal damage. Other complications include colicky abdominal pain, malaena, intussusception and joint involovement. Haematological investigations should be normal.

C28 FFTTF
Immunoglobulin G (IgG) has a molecular weight of 150 000 and is the most abundant immunoglobulin, particularly in the extravascular compartment. IgM is a pentamer with a molecular

weight of approximately 900 000 and is the first line defence against infection. IgM is also the most prominent class in the ABO blood group system, although clinically significant incompatibilities in the newborn period result from the passage of the more unusual IgG isoagglutinins across the placenta.

C29 FTFFT
Vaccines may be active or passive. Active vaccines can be divided into three main categories: (1) live attenuated, e.g. measles, mumps, rubella, BCG and oral polio (Sabin); (2) inactivated preparations, e.g. pertussis, typhoid, cholera, i.m. polio (Salk) and Hib; (3) toxoids, e.g. tetanus, diphtheria.

C30 FFTTF
This is a popular multiple choice subject but one where questions are likely to be particularly open to controversy, given conflicting reports relating to risks of transmission, both vertical and horizontal, and rapid developments in knowledge. Reports of the incidence of vertical transmission of HIV vary from around 13% to 65% and the virus has been identified in fetal tissue as early as 8 weeks' gestation. There is some evidence to suggest that the incidence may be reduced by delivery by caesarean section, but this does not seem to be universally agreed, and transmission in breast milk is also controversial. The virus is known to be present in breast milk, but the additional risk of infecting the infant is thought to be low, except in cases where the mother has received infected blood in the post-partum period and is therefore highly infectious during the breast-feeding period. Given the degree of uncertainty, it would be reasonable to counsel those at risk to use formula feeds.The role of antiviral therapy appears to be encouraging at reducing placental transmission. Laboratory diagnosis in infants is complicated by the presence of maternal antibodies, which may persist up to 18 or even 24 months and while a positive antigen test confirms the diagnosis a negative test does not exclude it.

C31 FFFTT
The incubation time of measles is 8–14 days and it is infectious for 7 days from the onset of the rash. Measles with a high fever is often complicated by convulsions and they are not indicative of encephalitis. Other complications include bronchitis, bronchopneumonia, suppurative otitis media, mastoiditis, severe oral inflammation, epistaxis, appendicitis and subacute sclerosing panencephalitis. The complications tend to be more severe where

malnutrition is present, and in some developing countries mortality is as high as 25%. Some degree of conjunctivitis and keratitis occurs in every case of measles. Selective suboccipital lymphadenopathy is a classical feature of rubella infection.

C32 FTFFT
Chloroquine when used once weekly for prophylaxis is generally well tolerated. However, if it is used for more than 3 years patients should undergo regular ophthalmic examination. Side effects are more serious if used at treatment levels for prolonged periods and these include electrocardiographic changes, retinal degeneration, bone marrow suppression and convulsions. Chloroquine is excreted in breast milk but the amount is insufficient to confer any benefit on the infant. Prophylaxis should be started 1 week prior to travel to an endemic region to allow detection of side effects and continued for 4 weeks after return.

C33 TTFTT
Congenital bone abnormalities such as a short femur or congenital dislocation of the hip result in a discrepancy of limb length. Soft tissue causes include haemangiomata (e.g. Klippel–Trenaunay syndrome), arteriovenous fistula and neurofibromatosis. Cerebral palsy and poliomyelitis cause shortening of the affected limb and Beckwith–Wiedemann and Russell–Silver syndromes are also associated with asymmetry. Chronic osteitis, which may result from tuberculosis, may interfere with bone growth.

C34 TFTFT
The most common complications of intrauterine growth retardation are hypothermia, hypoglycaemia and polycythaemia. These infants are less resilient to the stresses of labour, as they have relatively poor glycogen stores, are likely to have placental insufficiency and may have been exposed to chronic hypoxia *in utero*. Particularly careful monitoring is therefore required during labour. Small for gestational age infants are also said to be at increased risk of pulmonary haemorrhage, although this is a very rare complication. There is no significant increase in incidence of hyaline membrane disease in these infants or of infection in the newborn period.

C35 FTFTF
The risk of congenital rubella is high in the first and second trimesters (50–80% first trimester, 20–60% second trimester) but uncommon if maternal infection is in the third trimester. Common

clinical manifestations are intra-uterine growth retardation, microcephaly, deafness, cataracts and hepatosplenomegaly. Cerebral calcification is unusual, occurring more commonly in CMV and toxoplasmosis infection. Patent ductus arteriosus and peripheral pulmonary stenosis are the cardiac defects usually associated with congenital rubella. Vaccination of seronegative women should be delayed until after pregnancy because of the theoretical risks to the fetus associated with live vaccines.

C36 TTFTT
Oesophageal atresia is usually associated with a tracheo-oesophageal fistula but may occur in isolation. Many babies are also premature and of low birthweight. More than half the babies presenting with oesophageal atresia have associated congenital anomalies, commonly vertebral, anorectal, cardiac, tracheo-oesophageal fistula, renal and limb anomalies, particularly of the radius.These defects occur together sufficiently frequently to warrant joint consideration and have been given the acronyms VATER or VACTERAL.

C37 FTFTT
Common causes of tachypnoea with a primary respiratory cause presenting in the newborn period include respiratory distress syndrome (RDS), transient tachypnoea of the newborn, infection, pneumothorax, aspiration of meconium or milk, pulmonary hypoplasia (e.g. Potter's syndrome), and obstructive conditions (e.g. Pierre Robin syndrome, choanal atresia). Respiratory distress can also be secondary to extra-pulmonary pathology, for example congenital heart disease, high output cardiac failure in arteriovenous malformations (e.g. aneurysm of the vein of Galen), anaemia, metabolic acidosis and raised intracranial pressure. Wilson–Mikity syndrome presents in small preterm babies who did not have RDS. The onset is after the first week of life with gradual onset of tachypnoea, cyanosis and recurrent apnoea. Bronchopulmonary dysplasia is a chronic respiratory lung disease in babies who have required mechanical ventilation. The diagnosis is not usually made until the baby has been oxygen dependent for 28 days.

C38 FTTFF
Nocturnal enuresis affects 10–15% of 5 year olds, 5% of 10 year olds and 1–2% of 15 year olds, and tends to run in families. The sex ratio is equal in young children but males predominate among older children. Routine investigation should include examination

of urine to exclude urinary tract infection, diabetes insipidus and diabetes mellitus. In children with duplex collecting systems where the duplicated ureter(s) drain distal to the bladder neck, incontinence is likely to be worse on standing than lying down. In other cases of duplex, the incidence of enuresis should not be significantly different from the normal population.

C39 TFTTT
The majority of cases of HUS that occur follow a diarrhoeal prodrome, although a minority of cases follow respiratory illnesses. Recent epidemics have been associated with a verotoxin-producing strain of *E. coli*, serotype 0157:H7, but shigella dysentery may trigger some cases. Severe anaemia is usual, as is thrombocytopenia and neutrophilia. (See also A38.)

C40 FTFFT
Blood flow to the renal cortex is much greater than that to the medulla. Para-aminohippuric acid (PAH) is filtered by the glomeruli and secreted by the tubules, clearing 95% in one passage through the kidney. Clearance of PAH is lower in infants and it cannot therefore be used in this group to measure renal blood flow. The peritubular capillaries are at low pressure allowing fluid from the renal tubules to be absorbed. Hypoxia causes renal vasoconstriction.

C41 FTTFF
Complex partial seizures frequently originate in the temporal lobe which is why they used to be classed as temporal lobe epilepsy. They are characterized by alteration in behaviour, usually followed by abnormal motor activity, and may start with abnormal sensations, such as visual or auditory hallucinations or olfactory disturbance. Autonomic features are common, especially in infants, and may include flushing, sweating, pallor, nausea or vomiting. Awareness is affected to varying degrees during the seizure and there is usually a postictal phase of drowsiness. The EEG is frequently uninformative and there are usually no abnormalities to find between seizures. Febrile seizures are usually of the generalized tonic–clonic variety, although focal features are sometimes seen.

C42 TTFFT
Friedreich's ataxia is an autosomal recessive disorder. The main pathology is degeneration and demyelination of the spinocerebellar tracts, corticospinal pathways and posterior columns.

Cardiomyopathy occasionally presents before the ataxia, with angina, palpitations or dyspnoea. The ataxia is progressive, generally affecting the legs more than the arms. Plantar reflexes are extensor and ankle and knee jerks are usually absent. Posterior column involvement results in the loss of position and vibration sense. Other clinical features include dysarthria, scoliosis, pes cavus, nystagmus, optic atrophy, deafness and diabetes. Telangiectasia is seen in conjunction with ataxia telangiectasia but not Friedreich's ataxia.

C43 TTTTT
A complete list of the contents of breast milk is beyond the scope of this book, but its components may be subdivided into pure nutritional and immunological components. Nutritional components include casein, cholesterol, sodium, calcium, magnesium, vitamins A,C,D,E,K, thiamine and riboflavin. Non-nutritional or immunological components include lymphocytes, macrophages, lysozyme, secretory IgA and growth factors.

C44 TFFFT
Neuroblastomas arise from neural crest cells and occur with increased frequency in children with neurofibromatosis and Hirschsprung's disease; 85–90% of cases have raised catecholamine levels in blood and urine and the diagnosis must therefore rely on biopsy in the remainder. Additional findings include positive mIBG scan, elevated neuron-specific enolase, particularly in disseminated tumours, and ferritin, which is produced by the tumours in up to one-half of cases. Poor prognostic factors include age greater than 1 year at diagnosis, stage 3 and 4 tumours, abdominal primary, high serum ferritin and unfavourable cytogenetics.The finding of neuroblastoma tissue in autopsies performed on infants dying in the first few months of life from other causes suggests a high rate of spontaneous regression of neuroblastoma in this age group. Children, usually under 1 year of age, with stage 4S disease, characterized by localized primary tumour with dissemination limited to liver, skin and/or bone marrow, frequently recover with little or no treatment.

C45 FTFFT
Retinopathy of prematurity (ROP) is not clinically detectable until several weeks of age, and usually after 32 weeks post-menstrual age, although the environment in the first weeks of life is thought to be critical in its aetiology. The most important risk factors are prematurity, low birthweight and added oxygen

therapy. Fluctuations in transcutaneous Po_2 are also thought to be important. A significant proportion of low birthweight infants develop mild ROP (stages 1 and 2) which resolves spontaneously in most cases. Progression to stage 3 requires careful monitoring and may need treatment. The principle of treatment is to ablate the peripheral avascular retina thereby removing the stimulus for vessel growth and either laser or cryotherapy may be employed.

C46 FTFTT

Captopril is an angiotensin converting enzyme (ACE) inhibitor and leads to peripheral vasodilatation through reduction in angiotensin II levels. It is useful in patients with renin-dependent hypertension, such as those with renal parenchymal disease, but is contraindicated in patients with renal vascular disease, whose renal perfusion depends on an adequate renin drive. A lupus-like syndrome is more common in slow than fast acetylators and is seen with hydralazine, procainamide, phenytoin, ethosuximide and isoniazid. It is associated with HLA DR4. Nifedipine is rapidly absorbed from the stomach or the oral mucosa, hence its use in a sublingual preparation for the treatment of acute hypertension. Non-specific β-blockers such as propranolol, constrict bronchial smooth muscle. Phentolamine is a short acting α-adrenergic blocker and may be used in the diagnosis and acute treatment of phaeochromocytoma.

C47 TFTFF

Carbamazepine and phenobarbitone increase the rate of warfarin and aminophylline metabolism respectively. Cimetidine inhibits the metabolism of propranolol, this leading to increased levels. Probenicid may be used to potentiate the actions of penicillin by inhibiting its excretion and, by the same means, aspirin causes methotrexate levels to rise, thus enhancing its toxicity.

C48 FTTFF

Salbutamol is a selective $β_2$-agonist, relaxing bronchiolar and uterine muscle with relatively less $β_1$-effects on the heart. It stimulates membrane bound adenyl cyclase to increase intracellular cyclic AMP concentrations. Salbutamol can be administered orally, intravenously or by inhalation. Inhalation reduces but does not eliminate systemic side effects. Intravenous salbutamol is effective in the treatment of severe acute asthma but patients should be monitored closely for systemic side effects. Cardiovascular effects include positive inotropism and tachycardia. It also causes anxiety, tremor, nausea, sweating and the shift of potassium into cells, resulting in hypokalaemia.

C49 TTTFT
Ototoxicity from aminoglycoside antibiotics may present as vestibular dysfunction, auditory dysfunction or both. The incidence of ototoxicity is 2% for patients treated for less than 14 days. This incidence is increased with prolonged administration or high doses. Renal deficiency from any cause including birth asphyxia and old age increases toxicity. Renal function is impaired in more than 80% of patients treated with amphotericin B. Frusemide and mannitol also accentuate the ototoxic effects of aminoglycosides. Potassium levels do not have a recognized influence on aminoglycoside toxicity.

C50 TFFTT
Total body water accounts for 75% of the body weight at birth, and drops to 60% by a few years of age, corresponding to a reduction in extracellular water volume from 40% to 25%. The exact proportion is dependent on body fat. Intracellular water is fairly constant at 33%. Circulating blood volume is approximately 80 ml/kg, of which 45 ml/kg is plasma. Maintenance fluid requirements fall from 100 ml/kg/day in infancy to 40 ml/kg/day in adults. A useful formula for calculating requirements is as follows:

100 ml/kg/day for 1st 10 kg body weight
plus 50 ml/kg/day for 2nd 10 kg body weight
plus 20 ml/kg/day for remainder

Daily urine output is 1500 ml in an adult and 1–4 ml/kg in a small child. A urine output of less than 480 ml in a 20 kg child constitutes oliguria. Daily insensible fluid loss is approximately 30 ml/kg in infants, falling to 20 ml/kg in older children and 12 ml/kg in adults. More accurately it is calculated as 500 ml/m^2 of body surface area in older children and adults.

C51 TTFFT
The diagnosis of autism is dependent on three essential features: failure to develop social relationships; language abnormalities; and ritualistic or compulsive behaviour. It is three times more common in boys. Infants are often slow to smile and dislike physical contact. There is failure of eye contact and facial expression. Many children do not develop language and those that do, have abnormal features such as repetition of words and phrases. They often display rigid

patterns of play and have unusual preoccupations with figures such as learning timetables and dates. Seventy per cent of autistic children have intellectual retardation and only 5% of children have an IQ above 100. A quarter of adolescent autistics develop epilepsy.

C52 FTTFT
Causes of acute stridor include laryngotracheobronchitis (croup), due to infection by parainfluenza virus, adenovirus or respiratory syncytial virus, epiglottitis, bacterial tracheitis, inhalation of smoke or foreign body, diphtheria, acute angioneurotic oedema, retropharyngeal abscess and hypocalcaemia. Laryngomalacia (infantile or 'floppy' larynx) is one of the common causes of chronic stridor, along with acquired subglottic stenosis. Less common causes include congenital subglottic stenosis, haemangiomata, webs, cysts, laryngeal clefts, vascular rings, tracheal stenosis and vocal cord palsy.

C53 TFTFT
The sweat test remains the major diagnostic tool for the confirmation of CF, despite the recognition of the CF gene and some of its mutations. Not all mutations of the gene are yet identified, and most centres only routinely look for the most common gene defects. Gene analysis can detect 75–85% of homozygotes. The most common defect is the δF508 gene defect with an incidence of 67% in the CF population. The incidence of the CF phenotype in the UK is approximately 1 in 2500, but it is extremely rare in non-caucasians populations.

C54 FFTTT
Tidal volume corresponds to normal breathing. If a maximal inspiration is followed by maximal expiration, the resulting exhaled volume is known as the vital capacity. However, some gas remains in the lung after maximal expiration and this is the residual volume. The volume of gas in the lung after a normal tidal breath is the functional residual capacity. The total lung capacity is the vital capacity plus the residual volume. Neither the functional residual capacity nor the residual volume can be measured with a simple spirometer. They can be calculated using a gas dilutional technique or using a body plethysmograph.

C55 TTTTT
Obesity is usually due to excessive eating but may result from reduced energy output due to physical handicap. There are many syndromes associated with obesity including Laurence–Moon–Biedl,

the features of which also include polydactyly, retinitis pigmentosa and hypogonadism. Prader–Willi syndrome presents with neonatal hypotonia and initially poor feeding, obesity not usually developing until the second year of life due to excessive eating. Endocrine and metabolic causes of obesity include hypopituitarism, Cushing's syndrome, insulinoma and pseudohypoparathyroidism. Drugs which increase the appetite and cause excessive weight gain include clonazepam, sodium valproate and prolonged corticosteroid therapy.

C56 TTFFF
A type I error is a hypothesis which is rejected by a significance test when it is true, and a type II error is a hypothesis which is accepted when it is false. The standard error of the mean is the standard deviation of the sampling distribution of the mean. It is used to give an indication of the adequacy of the sample mean as an estimator of the population mean. It equates to the population standard deviation divided by the square root of the number in the sample, for a continuous distribution. Some adjustment is required when the population is finite, but the principles are the same. Probability is denoted by the letter P and may assume a value from 0 to 1. $P = 1$ means that the event always occurs and $P = 0$ means that it will never occur.

C57 FFTFT
Inappropriate antidiuretic hormone secretion is most commonly seen in neonates in association with birth asphyxia, respiratory distress syndrome or intraventricular haemorrhage. In older children it is associated with meningitis, encephalitis, pneumonia or cerebral tumours. It commonly occurs for a few days following a general anaesthetic. It results in water retention, hypo-osmolality and dilutional hyponatraemia. Urine is concentrated and there is usually no oedema. Treatment is by water restriction but, if this fails, drug treatment may be necessary and frusemide with sodium replacement may be effective for this purpose.

C58 FTTFT
There are numerous causes of visual defects which may involve any part of the visual pathway from the cornea through to the visual cortex. Prenatal causes include congenital rubella, cytomegalovirus, toxoplasmosis and maternal treatment with phenothiazines and warfarin. Retinopathy of prematurity is closely related to gestational age, and premature infants are more likely to have myopia and squints. Cerebral palsy, hydrocephalus

and craniosynostosis, including Apert's syndrome are all risk factors and galactosaemia is associated with cataracts. Children with juvenile chronic arthritis, particularly the pauciarticular variety, are at risk of uveitis (iridocyclitis) and should therefore be screened regularly. Isolated conjunctival haemorrhages in neonates may look dramatic but parents may be reassured that vision will be unaffected. Henoch–Schönlein purpura is not associated with visual complications.

C59 TFFFF

Headaches which are likely to be non-organic in origin characteristically occur daily, with little variation in intensity, or are associated with particular environments; for example, children with a tendency towards school refusal may have symptoms restricted to term time. Other associated symptoms, such as abdominal pain, and behavioural and emotional changes are frequently seen and there is often a positive family history. Recurrent abdominal pain occurs in up to 10% of children and is non-organic in 90% of cases. The pain is characteristically diffuse or periumbilical, restricted to the daytime, associated with pain elsewhere and with normal findings on physical exmaination and investigation. Non-organic headaches and abdominal pain may sometimes be classified as somatoform disorders, characterized by symptoms which may suggest organic disease, although there is no other evidence of such disease. The subject is consciously unaware of the underlying problem and is therefore not malingering. Other complaints include visual problems, paralyses, seizures and limb pain. Backache is an unusual presentation of psychological disturbance in childhood and should therefore be taken seriously and investigated thoroughly. Pseudo-seizures, which are simulations of seizures by patients, occur more commonly in epileptics than non-epileptics and particularly in those with behavioural or emotional problems. They can be extremely difficult to differentiate from genuine seizures but certain features serve as pointers; pseudo-seizures tend to be more gradual in onset and do not occur when the patient is asleep or alone, they are more likely to have unusual features and may be suspected when previously effective treatment suddenly appears to lose its efficacy.

C60 TFTFT

The normal cardiac action potential results from changes in the permeability of the cardiac cell membranes to sodium, potassium and calcium during phases 0 to 4. Phase 4 is the resting phase; contractile cells have a constant resting potential around $-90\,\text{mV}$

until activated, but the pacemaker cells exhibit spontaneous phase 4 depolarization until a threshold of approximately –70 mV is reached. At this level, a rapid influx of sodium occurs through channels causing depolarization to a peak of 20 mV. This is followed by repolarization in phases 1, 2 and 3.

Practice examination D   Answers

D1 FTFFT
The posterior interosseous nerve is the deep terminal branch of the radial nerve and may be damaged following dislocation of the elbow or supracondylar fracture of the humerus. It supplies abductor pollicis longus, supinator and all of the extensors of the hand and forearm except for extensor carpi radialis longus. Branches of the median nerve supply pronator teres and pronator quadratus, in the latter case via the anterior interosseous branch. The posterior interosseous nerve supplies a number of the joints of the forearm and hand, mostly shared with other nerves, and does not have a sensory distribution. The loss of sensation resulting from more proximal radial nerve damage is limited to a small area on the lateral aspect of the dorsum of the hand.

D2 FFTFT
Hypertension and hypokalaemia coexist when there is an increased mineralocorticoid drive. Causes include exogenous steroid administration, adrenal adenoma or carcinoma, a proportion of cases of congenital adrenal hyperplasia caused by 11β-hydroxylase deficiency and secondary hyperaldosteronism, usually the consequence of increased renin production, such as in renal artery stenosis. Addison's disease leads to adrenocortical hypofunction with resulting hyperkalaemia and Bartter's syndrome is associated with hyperaldosteronism and normotension. 21α-Hydroxylase deficiency is classically associated with salt wasting, hyperkalaemia and hypotension although, in some cases, mineralocorticoid biosynthesis is intact.

D3 FTTFT
Conditions other than cystic fibrosis associated with raised sweat electrolytes are rare and the levels are usually less elevated. They include adrenal insufficiency, ectodermal dysplasia, hypothyroidism, familial hypoparathyroidism, nephrogenic diabetes insipidus, glycogen storage disease type 1, anorexia nervosa and severe malnutrition.

D4 TFFFT
Heart failure in childhood most commonly presents in the first few months of life as a result of congenital heart disease. Poor feeding, pallor, restlessness and rapid breathing may be noted by the parents and sweating is often profuse, as the only mechanism by which the infant can maintain body temperature in the presence of high metabolic rate and reduced peripheral perfusion. The most common signs are tachycardia, tachypnoea and

hepatomegaly. A heart rate over 180 beats per minute is supportive of the diagnosis of heart failure, but supraventricular tachycardia is unlikely unless the rate rises above 200. Jugular venous pressure is not a useful sign in infants, due to the shortness of their necks, lack of cooperation and difficulty in immobilizing the area of interest.

D5 TFTTF
Cardiologists have differing opinions as to which lesions should be covered by antibiotics and, although they would probably all agree to cover those at high risk of infective endocarditis, prophylaxis for those at low risk is more controversial. The haemodynamic situation most likely to predispose to infective endocarditis is a high pressure jet into a lower pressure system through a narrow orifice with turbulence. Therefore a ventricular septal defect is much more likely to become infected than an atrial septal defect. Lesions at highest risk of infective endocarditis include aortic valve disease (bicuspid or rheumatic), mitral valve disease, coarctation, a patent ductus arteriosus (PDA), ventricular septal defects and prosthetic valves. There is an increased risk in patients with hypertrophic cardiomyopathy and subaortic stenosis. Infective endocarditis is very rare in atrial septal defects and a divided PDA. It should be remembered that a previously apparently normal heart valve can become infected.

D6 FTFFF
The revised Jones criteria requires two major, or one major and two minor criteria, in addition to evidence of streptococcal infection. Major criteria are carditis, polyarthritis, chorea, erythema marginatum and subcutaneous nodules. Minor criteria include previous rheumatic fever, arthralgia, fever, raised ESR, leucocytosis and a prolonged PR interval.

D7 TFFTT
The second heart sound is due to closure of the aortic and pulmonary valves. The aortic component is heard first and is louder than the pulmonary component. It occurs at the end of systole and coincides with the end of the T wave of the electrocardiogram. The loudness of the second heart sound is determined by the rate of decrease of ventricular pressure at the end of systole. It is therefore increased in pulmonary or systemic hypertension. The second heart sound is widely split in right bundle branch block, deep inspiration, mitral regurgitation and ventricular septal defects. There is reversed splitting in left bundle branch

block and aortic stenosis and fixed splitting in atrial septal defect.
There is a single second sound in Fallot's tetralogy, severe
pulmonary stenosis, severe aortic stenosis, pulmonary atresia and
large ventricular septal defects.

D8 FFFTT
Nappy rash due to candidiasis characteristically involves the
inguinal folds, unlike that due to chemical irritation. Harlequin
colour change, where one half of the body becomes episodically
erythematous, is seen mainly in premature neonates as a consequence of immaturity of the autonomic control of peripheral
vascular tone. It usually resolves within a few days of birth and is
not associated with any significant cardiovascular or neurological
abnormality. Port wine stains do not resolve spontaneously but
may be reduced in size and intensity by laser treatment. Epidermolysis bullosa has a large number of variants, many of which
present from birth with blistering at sites of trauma. Erythema
toxicum usually appears between 24 and 48 h of age but may
occur from birth to 14 days.

D9 FTFTF
A normal 6 month old would be expected to hold his head up well
and, in the prone position, support his head and shoulders on two
hands. Most would be sitting with minimal support but very few
would be crawling. This may start as early as 6 months and most
crawl by 9 months but some infants never crawl, preferring to
bottom shuffle. The stepping reflex should be lost by 2–3 months.
The pincer grasp does not develop until 9 or 10 months so a 6-
month-old infant would be expected to use an ulnar grasp to pick
up objects. Infants should still to their mothers' voice from 3
months and shyness with strangers usually develops from 5 or 6
months. All objects tend to go straight to the mouth at around 6
months and this habit continues until about 12 months of age.

D10 TTFFT
The most common cause of speech delay is intellectual retardation including cerebral palsy, Down's syndrome, untreated
hypothyroidism and untreated phenylketonuria (PKU). In an
otherwise normal, healthy child there is often a family history of
delayed speech. Deafness is an important cause, and all children
with speech problems should have a careful hearing assessment.
Social causes such as emotional deprivation or child abuse
commonly lead to delayed speech. Twins are often late to speak,
the cause of which is unclear. Tongue tie probably causes no

speech problems at all, and certainly should not cause delay. Subacute sclerosing panencephalitis (SSPE) does not usually occur until 5–10 years after infection with measles and will lead to speech regression rather than delay.

D11 TFTFT
Testis determining factor, encoded by the SRY gene on the Y chromosome, stimulates the undifferentiated gonad to develop into a testis. In its absence, ovarian tissue develops. Müllerian inhibiting factor (MIF) is secreted by the Sertoli cells of the testes. It inhibits the differentiation of the Müllerian ducts into uterus and fallopian tubes. Testosterone, secreted by the Leydig cells, maintains the Wolffian duct and promotes development of the male internal genitalia, whereas the role of dihydrotestosterone is in the development of the external genitalia.

D12 TFTFF
Acute lead poisoning is rare, but chronic lead poisoning is more frequent. In childhood, chronic poisoning is typically due to ingestion of lead-containing paint in old homes or drinking water from lead pipes. Ingestion of car battery fluid may cause acute lead poisoning. Lead partially inhibits haem synthetase resulting in very high levels of free erythrocyte protoporphyrin and urinary δ aminolaevulinic acid. Poisoning may lead to a Fanconi-type renal tubular acidosis but is not associated with nephrogenic diabetes insipidus. Other features of lead poisoning include anaemia, constipation, abdominal pain, anorexia, nausea, dense metaphyseal bands at the growing ends of long bones, peripheral nerve lesions, seizures and reduced consciousness.

D13 FFFTT
Three per cent of normal children fall below the 3rd centile for height. This alone is therefore not an indication for further investigation, unless height is falling away from the centile. Centiles for growth velocity do not correspond precisely to centiles for absolute height as the difference between the height centiles widens with increasing age. For example, while a child on the 50th centile will stay on their centile if their growth velocity is also on the 50th centile, persistent growth velocity below the 25th centile, while not necessarily abnormal, will lead to a gradual fall off in height away from the 3rd centile (this is a popular trap set by examiners, although routine measurement of growth velocity may become obsolete with increased use of cross-sectional charts showing additional centile points from 0.4 to 99.6). Predicted

height is based on the midpoint between the parental height centiles and, in 95% of cases, will fall within 8.5 cm of this height. Exercise stress tests are only useful to exclude growth hormone deficiency. A subnormal response is not diagnostic and needs to be followed by a pharmacological stimulation test.

D14 FFFTT
In addition to the three zones found in adults, the fetal adrenal has a distinct fetal zone which secretes weak androgens, metabolized by the placenta. Cortisol is secreted by the zona glomerulosa, aldosterone from the zona fasciculata and androgens from the zona reticularis. Levels of cortisol peak between 0400 and 0800 h, and are lowest between 2000 h and midnight. In females, pubic hair development depends on adrenal androgen production but, in males, the adrenal makes a small contribution to the circulating androgen pool compared with gonadal output, especially from puberty onwards. Without glucocorticoids, which are essential for water, carbohydrate, protein and fat metabolism, and mineralo-corticoids, essential for the maintenance of blood pressure, the ability to respond to even minor noxious stimuli is lost.

D15 TTFTF
Atrial natriuretic factor (ANF) is synthesized in the cardiac atria in concentrations linearly related to right and left atrial pressures and also to atrial diameter. It produces an increase in urine volume and sodium excretion primarily by increasing the glomerular filtration rate. It is a potent vasodilator and antago-nizes the release and effects of renin, aldosterone and antidiuretic hormone.

D16 FTTTT
Thyroid stimulating hormone (TSH) is secreted by the anterior pituitary. Its secretion is controlled by thyrotrophin releasing hormone from the hypothalamus, as well as negative feedback from circulating thyroid hormones. Thyrotrophin releasing hormone secretion is increased by exposure to the cold and decreased by sympathetic nervous stimulation. The hypothalamus can inhibit TSH by secreting somatostatin which also inhibits growth hormone secretion. TSH increases the activities of the thyroid glandular cells, mostly via the activation of cyclic AMP. The most important early effect of TSH is to increase the proteolysis of thyroglobulin, releas-ing thyroid hormones into the blood. It increases the uptake of iodide by the thyroid gland, increases the size and number of thyroid cells and stimulates the activity of these cells.

D17 TTTTF

Growth failure is the most common extraintestinal complication of Crohn's disease and may be the presenting feature. Non-erosive arthritis, usually of the large peripheral joints, occurs frequently and reflects the level of disease activity. Ankylosing spondylitis occurs more commonly in patients who are HLA B27 positive and is unrelated to bowel disease activity. Ocular complications may occur in approximately 10% of patients, uveitis being the most common, but there is a risk of progression to cataract formation and glaucoma, and chorioretinitis, episcleritis, corneal lesions and granulomatous conjunctivitis are also recognized. Other manifestations include hepatic abnormalities and skin lesions, including pyoderma gangrenosum, which is more commonly associated with ulcerative colitis, and erythema nodosum.

D18 TFFTF

Following the breakdown of red blood cells bilirubin is formed via compounds including biliverdin. Bilirubin is transported in the blood tightly bound to albumin. It is conjugated in the liver with glucuronic acid, under the influence of glucuronyl transferase, to create a water soluble compound which is secreted in the bile. The bilirubin is broken down in the liver and gut to urobilinogen and stercobilinogen which are both colourless. These are oxidized to urobilin and stercobilin which give the faeces a brown colour. Some of the urobilinogen is reabsorbed in the small intestine. Most of this is re-excreted via the liver into the gut, but approximately 5% is excreted by the kidneys in the urine. Gilbert's syndrome is a partial deficiency of glucuronyl transferase.

D19 FTFFT

Gastric acid is secreted by parietal cells. Secretion depends on stimulation of receptors by histamine, acetylcholine (via the vagus nerve) and gastrin. Vagotomy reduces secretion but does not abolish it because local factors persist. Hydrogen chloride is necessary to split pepsinogen to form pepsin. Once formed pepsin is only active under acid conditions and hydrogen chloride is therefore essential for protein digestion to occur in the stomach. Secretin stimulates pancreatic secretion and opposes the effects of gastrin.

D20 TTFTT

Chronic duodenal ulcers are uncommon throughout childhood and particularly rare before the age of 5 years, but are seen more often than chronic gastric ulcers. There is often a positive family history and boys are affected slightly more frequently than girls. Barium meal has a relatively poor sensitivity and endoscopy is the investigation of choice. This also allows for biopsies to look for *Helicobacter pylori*. Non-organic abdominal pain accounts for the majority of recurrent abdominal pain in childhood.

D21 TFTTT

Non-disjunction of chromosome 21, where the paired chromosomes fail to move to opposite poles duing meiosis, leading to trisomy, accounts for approximately 95% of cases of Down's syndrome. Duodenal atresia, though rare, is the major gastrointestinal malformation associated with Down's syndrome, which accounts for 30% of cases. More than 50% have significant hearing difficulties and approximately one third of adults will ultimately be affected with Alzheimer's disease. The relatively poor prognosis in leukaemia associated with Down's syndrome appears to be due to increased susceptibility to infection and myelotoxicity. Levels of alphafetoprotein and unconjugated oestriol are lower and human chorionic gonadotrophin higher than normal in maternal serum, and these are frequently used as a basis for screening.

D22 FFFTT

An X-linked condition or phenotype which is regularly expressed in heterozygotes can be described as dominant. All of the daughters and none of the sons of affected males are affected. The pattern of inheritance through affected females is no different from the autosomal dominant mode of inheritance. The best known example is vitamin D-resistant or familial hypophosphataemic rickets. The phenotype in females affected by X-linked dominant conditions is frequently less severe than in males, and ornithine transcarbamylase deficiency is an example of this. Rare genetic defects which are only expressed phenotypically in females are likely to be X-linked dominant conditions that are lethal to males *in utero*; Rett syndrome is one such example. Becker muscular dystrophy is X-linked recessive, Tay–Sachs disease autosomal recessive and familial hypercholesterolaemia autosomal dominant.

D23 FFTTT

In an autosomal recessive condition, only homozygotes for the abnormal allele are affected but heterozygotes are carriers. Affected individuals therefore have parents who are both carriers but neither parent is phenotypically affected. If a parent is affected, all of the offspring will be carriers but none of them affected, unless the other parent is also a carrier. On average, half of the offspring of two carriers will be carriers themselves, one quarter affected and one quarter neither affected nor carriers. Thus if the carrier rate is 1 in 50, the chance of two carriers reproducing is 1 in 2500, and the number of affected individuals 1 in 10 000 of the population. A union between related individuals, who are likely to be carriers for the same recessive conditions, is more likely to produce affected children.

D24 FTTTT
Maternal diabetes, thyrotoxicosis, congenital adrenal hyperplasia, chromosome abnormalities (trisomies 13, 18 and 21) and any causes of placental insufficiency lead to increased intrauterine erythropoiesis. Passive causes of polycythaemia may result from materno-fetal or twin-to-twin transfusions, delayed cord clamping or unattended delivery. Congenital rubella is a cause of thrombocytopenia.

D25 FFTTF
Von Willebrand disease is an autosomal dominant condition. Since the development of sensitive methods for detecting its mildest forms, it has been claimed by some to be the commonest congenital bleeding disorder. It results from a functional abnormality in factor VIII, leading to failure of platelets to adhere to the subendothelial matrix. It presents with a history of excessive bruising or bleeding, either mucosal or following surgery or trauma. Findings include a prolonged bleeding time and usually prolonged partial thromboplastin time, with low levels of factor VIII:C and factor VIII related antigen, and failure of ristocetin to induce platelet aggregation. Antenatal diagnosis may be performed by enzyme assay of fetal blood samples or DNA analysis. Treatment of mild and moderate bleeds may involve the use of the posterior pituitary hormone analogue DDAVP, which releases stored von Willebrand factor and provides a haemostatic effect for approximately 4 h. For more severe bleeds, this approach is insufficient and factor VIII concentrates are required.

D26 FTTTT
Fanconi's anaemia is an autosomal dominant disorder which may present with aplastic anaemia, leukaemia, leukopenia or thrombocytopenia. It is associated with hyperpigmentation, microcephaly, thumb abnormalities, renal anomalies, ear abnormalities and

mental retardation. Hereditary spherocytosis and sickle cell disease are disorders of the red cell and should not influence the white cell count, although both cause splenomegaly in early childhood. Hurler syndrome is a mucopolysaccharidosis; its features include developmental delay with eventual regression, hepatosplenomegaly, course facies and umbilical and inguinal hernias. It is associated with an increased incidence of respiratory and middle ear infections which may affect the white cell count, but the count is neither raised nor depressed in normal circumstances.

D27 TTFFF

C reactive protein (CRP) is an acute phase protein, produced by the liver following cytokine stimulation, in response to activation of the inflammatory process by bacterial products or tissue damage. It rises in cases of necrotizing enterocolitis but not following intraventricular haemorrhage. During bacterial infection, the CRP rises rapidly, over hours, and has a positive predictive value of between 50 and 60%. Levels usually return to normal within 96 h once the stimulus to its production has been removed. CRP has a molecular weight of greater than 100 kDa, which makes transplacental passage unlikely, and this conclusion is borne out by biochemical and clinical studies. Interleukin-6 (IL-6) does cross the placenta and could therefore theoretically produce a transient CRP response in the newborn infant, but its half-life is short.

D28 FTTFF

There are three basic interferons – alpha, beta and gamma. Interferon gamma (INF-γ) is produced mainly by T lymphocytes. Although it has some antiviral activity, it is primarily a cytokine concerned with modulating immune responses. It has potent phagocyte activating effects not seen with INF-α or INF-β and is used as an adjunct therapy with antibiotics to reduce the incidence of serious infections in patients with chronic granulomatous disease. INF-α and INF-β share a common cell surface receptor, but INF-γ is structurally poorly related and binds to its own specific receptor. INF-α and INF-β are produced by peripheral blood mononuclear cells and fibroblasts respectively, as a response to the presence of viruses and certain intracellular bacteria. They have potent antiviral activity, have enhancing effects on some immune mechanisms and are potent inhibitors of normal and malignant cell growth. IFN-α is active against some human malignancies and uses include the treatment of hairy cell leukaemia, recurrent or metastatic renal cell carcinoma and AIDS-related Kaposi's sarcoma.

D29 TTTTF
Systemic lupus erythematosus, acute nephritis, membranoproliferative glomerulonephritis, Gram-negative sepsis, acute pancreatitis and acute vasculitis are all associated with complement
consumption. Hereditary angio-oedema is due to deficiency of C1
esterase inhibitor. Levels of C4 are persistently low due to excessive consumption.

D30 TTFFF
In children with HIV, tests of immune competence show that
polyclonal hypergammaglobulinaemia is an early finding, and high
levels of IgG may coexist with subclass deficiencies. B cell
dysfunction is often detected before T cell abnormalities and low
CD4+:CD8+ ratios are seen relatively late. Less than 4% of
children with AIDS have Kaposi's sarcoma, a markedly lower
incidence than in infected homosexual men. Major side effects
following immunization of HIV infected children have not been
encountered and routine immunizations, apart from BCG, should
be given. In children with symptomatic HIV infection, antibodies
to the vaccines should be monitored, since responses to them may
be impaired, and passive immunization may need to be considered. Persistence of the p24 antigen and loss of p24 antibody are
indicators of poor prognosis, along with age less than 1 year at
diagnosis, pneumocystis pneumonia infection and the presence of
a number of cellular and serological markers.

D31 FTTTT
Typhoid fever is caused by infection with *Salmonella typhi*, usually
as a result of ingestion of contaminated food or water. *S.
typhimurium* causes enteritis, or salmonellosis, as opposed to
enteric fever, which includes typhoid and paratyphoid. Clinical
features include a swinging pyrexia, influenza-like symptoms,
cough, drowsiness, abdominal pain, diarrhoea or constipation, and
a macular rash or 'rose spots', from which the organism may be
cultured. A bradycardia, relative to the pyrexia is frequently
present in adults but not usually in young children. Antibiotic
choices may include amoxicillin, trimethoprim, co-trimoxazole or
chloramphenicol, depending on sensitivities.

D32 FTTTF
Mumps infection has an incubation period of 14–18 days and is
infectious from 6 days before to 4 days after salivary gland
swelling; 30–40% of infections are asymptomatic. In symptomatic
cases, the parotid is the gland most commonly affected by swelling

and this is frequently unilateral or asymmetrical. Amylase is often slightly raised even in the absence of pancreatitis which is a very rare complication of mumps. Orchitis is unusual before puberty but is seen in up to 20% of cases in adolescent males and is usually unilateral. Meningoencephalitis may be the presenting feature and polyneuritis, trigeminal or facial neuritis and retrobulbar optic neuritis have also occasionally been noted. Other rare complications include myocarditis, mild disturbances of hepatic enzymes and arthritis. Killed vaccines against mumps have only short-term benefit but the attenuated live vaccine, now widely used, leads to 95% seroconversion.

D33 FFFFT
Metaphysial tenderness is typical of acute osteomyelitis, the likely diagnosis in this case. Septic arthritis presents as a hot, tender joint with effusion. Plain X-ray changes in bone take 7–10 days to develop, although soft tissue changes will be evident much earlier, and since the differential diagnosis includes fracture, an X-ray is justified. More than 80% of acute childhood bone and joint infections are caused by *Staphylococcus aureus*. Where a confident clinical diagnosis of acute infection can be made, antibiotic treatment should not be delayed once blood cultures have been taken. However, in chronic cases, diagnosis should precede treatment. Typical cases of acute osteomyelitis and septic arthritis have an excellent prognosis in the developed world, given prompt and appropriate treatment.

D34 TFTFT
Cystic fibrosis occurs with an incidence of approximately 1 in 2500. The reported incidence of hypospadias varies between 1:150 and 1:300, giving 6–12 cases per year in this population. Perinatal mortality includes stillbirths after 28 weeks' gestation and deaths in the first week of life. Haemorrhagic disease of the newborn is extremely rare. A British survey in 1988/90 found its incidence to range from about 1 per million births for infants given intramuscular vitamin K prophylaxis to 1 per 10 000 for the minority given no prophylaxis. The incidence of natural twins is approximately 1:80 but use of fertility programmes increases this figure.

D35 TTTFT
In the course of withdrawal from *in utero* narcotic exposure, wakefulness, irritability, tremulousness, temperature variability, tachypnoea, hyperactivity, high-pitched cry, hyperacusis, hypertonia, diarrhoea, disorganized suck, respiratory distress,

rhinorrhoea, rub marks, apnoea, weight loss or failure to gain adequate weight, alkalosis, lacrimation (mnemonic WITHDRAWAL), as well as vomiting, hiccoughs, seizures and jerking, sneezing, yawning, and photophobia, may all be seen.

D36 TTTFT
Bile stained vomiting suggests the presence of a mechanical or functional bowel obstruction distal to the ampulla of Vater. Causes include developmental abnormalities of the gut, such as atresias of the duodenum, jejunum and ileum, and malrotation with volvulus. Necrotizing enterocolitis is primarily a disease of the very low birthweight preterm infant and most commonly occurs in the first week of life. Other conditions which may present with bilious vomiting include meconium ileus, secondary to cystic fibrosis, strangulated inguinal hernia and Hirschsprung's disease, although this is more likely to be picked up as a result of delay in the passage of meconium.

D37 TFTTT
Polyhydramnios occurs in 1–2% of pregnancies and is often associated with multiple pregnancy or maternal diabetes. Congenital abnormalities associated with polyhydramnios include oesophageal atresia, duodenal atresia, neural tube defects, neuromuscular disorders, hydrops and diaphragmatic hernia. Often no cause can be identified. Potter's syndrome is caused by oligohydramnios, usually the consequence of bilateral renal agenesis, and results in facial dysmorphism, pulmonary hypoplasia and limb deformities.

D38 TFTFT
Energy intake should be maximized in renal failure to prevent the use of nitrogen sources as fuel, thereby contributing to uraemia, and protein intake should be carefully controlled. Calorie supplementation is frequently employed. Renal osteodystrophy, resulting from impaired 25-hydroxycholecalciferol metabolism, is characterized by reduced calcium absorption and hyperphosphataemia. The latter is controlled by a combination of dietary phosphate restriction and administration of phosphate binders. Potassium restriction is less important in chronic than acute renal failure, but potassium binges should be avoided. In nephrotic syndrome, gentle salt restriction is often advocated, although it may exacerbate the hypovolaemic state, whereas a high salt intake may worsen oedema. A normal 'no added salt' diet is probably the most appropriate. Adequate protein intake is essential, but

despite the glomerular loss of albumin, nephrotics do not tolerate high protein intakes, particularly if unwell.

D39 TTFTF
Postinfectious glomerulonephritis typically occurs 10 days after a Group A streptococcal infection of the nasopharynx or skin, most commonly in school age children, but any age can be affected. With the reduction in number of cases of poststreptococcal glomerulonephritis in developed countries, other bacterial and viral causes are increasingly being recognized, including pneumococcal, staphylococcal, salmonella and mycoplasma species, coxsackie, ECHO, Epstein Barr and influenza viruses. Clinical features include nonspecific symptoms of malaise, smoky urine, oliguria, oedema, often starting on the face, and hypertension. Investigations may reveal renal impairment of varying severity, haematuria with casts and, in particularly oedematous cases, evidence of pleural effusion or rarely even pulmonary oedema on the chest X-ray. Complement is reduced and antistreptolysin O (ASO) titre usually raised, although the latter may not be affected by skin infections, in which cases anti-DNAase B titres should also be measured. Specific treatment can be limited to penicillin for 10 days, and supportive treatment which may include anti-hypertensives and, in only the most severe cases, dialysis. The outlook is excellent in most cases and renal biopsy is therefore only indicated for those cases who do not respond to treatment, or have progressive disease.

D40 TFFFT
Up to 10% of children with facial (VIIth nerve) palsy have hypertension, and a significant minority of children with hypertension develop facial palsy. Other causes of unilateral lower motor neuron facial palsy include Lyme disease, leukaemia, brain stem tumours, middle ear disease and birth trauma. In dystrophia myotonica, facioscapulohumoral dystrophy, congenital myopathies and Guillain–Barré syndrome, the damage is more commonly bilateral. Upper motor neuron lesions spare the upper part of the face due to dual innervation, and these may be the result of intracranial pathology, including cerebral hemisphere tumours. Facial palsy of undetermined cause, known as Bell's palsy, is in most cases thought to be a parainfectious mononeuritis, occurring 1–3 weeks after a viral illness. It is due to demyelination and oedema of the nerve. Provided that more sinister causes can be excluded, corticosteroids or ACTH may have useful immunosuppressant and anti-inflammatory effects, but are seldom effective unless started within 72 h of the onset.

D41 FFFTT
The CSF is secreted by the choroid plexus in the lateral ventricles and should be colourless. The normal CSF pressure is 5–15 cm CSF with the patient recumbent. Raised CSF protein is found in Gullain–Barré syndrome, meningitis, multiple sclerosis and hypothyroidism.

D42 FTTFF
Febrile convulsions are common, occurring in 3% of children. They usually occur between the ages of 6 months and 5 years. Recurrence occurs in one-third of cases but only rarely will a child have more than one convulsion in the same illness. Sometimes the seizures will be unilateral (4–18%), or prolonged (4–30%). These seizures are said to be complicated or complex and have a higher incidence of subsequent epilepsy. The mild pyrexia sometimes associated with teething does not cause febrile convulsions.

D43 FTFFF
Vitamin D is produced in the skin as cholecalciferol. This is hydrolysed in the liver to 25-hydroxycalciferol and then by the kidney to 1, 25-dihydroxycholecalciferol. Ileal disease or resection leads to decreased absorption of vitamin B_{12}. Renal disease results in vitamin D deficiency.

D44 TTTFT
Leukaemia and lymphoma are recognized complications of both Bruton's disease, or X-linked agammaglobulinaemia, and Wiskott–Aldrich syndrome. Beckwith–Wiedemann syndrome predisposes to Wilms' tumour, adrenal carcinoma and hepatoblastoma and neurofibromatosis to sarcoma, phaeochromocytoma, leukaemia and neural tumours. Other inherited conditions with increased incidence of malignancy include tuberous sclerosis, von Hippel–Lindau's syndrome, familial polyposis coli, ataxia telangiectasia, Fanconi's disease, haemochromatosis, galactosaemia, Wilson's syndrome, α-1 antitrypsin deficiency, multiple exostosis and fibro-osseous dysplasia.

D45 TFFFT
There are very few drugs that are absolutely contraindicated in breast feeding. Cytotoxics, radiopharmaceuticals, lithium, immunosuppressants, phenindione and ergotamine are of sufficient concern to avoid altogether. Many others are known to be secreted in breast milk but, in general, in insufficient quantities to cause harm to the infant.

D46 TFFTT
Amiodarone is an effective anti-arrhythmic agent, particularly for
supraventricular tachycardia, but its long half-life and adverse
effects warrant caution in its use and careful monitoring. It can
be given once daily but may take several weeks to build up to an
effective dose and side effects may persist for some months after
it is discontinued. Its most important toxic effects involve the
thyroid, frequent skin photosensitivity, and the cornea, where
asymptomatic deposits are extremely common, necessitating
regular monitoring by slit lamp examination. Other effects include
pulmonary fibrosis, hepatitis, peripheral neuropathy and
occasional cerebellar toxicity.

D47 FFTTT
Renal excretion contributes to some extent for the removal from
the body of most antibiotics and an up-to-date formulary should
be consulted before prescribing any drug to a patient with
impaired renal function. Drugs of the penicillin and aminoglycoside groups are mostly excreted unchanged in the urine. Of the
tetracycline group, doxycycline and minocycline are mainly
metabolized but the remainder are excreted in the urine 40–60%
unchanged. Erythromycin and metronidazole are not excreted in
the urine to a significant extent, being mostly metabolized by the
liver.

D48 TFFTF
Chemotherapy associated with a high emetogenic potential
include cisplatin, doxorubicin, daunorubicin, high dose cyclophos-
phamide and high dose carboplatin. Vincristine, vinblastine and
methotrexate are generally not associated with severe nausea or
vomiting. Ondansetron is an affective antiemetic to administer
prior to commencing chemotherapy with the more emetic agents,
while domperidone, metoclopramide and prochlorperazine are
suitable for use with less emetic chemotherapy.

D49 FFTFF
Drugs taken orally are mostly absorbed from the small intestine
into the portal venous blood and pass through the liver prior to
entering the systemic circulation. Some drugs undergo extensive
hepatic or first pass metabolism and are therefore ineffective by
this route. Drugs administered high into the rectum are absorbed
into the superior haemorrhoidal veins and pass to the portal
system to undergo first pass metabolism, whereas those administered low avoid passing to the liver before entering the systemic

circulation. The sublingual route also bypasses the liver. The amount of a drug absorbed following oral administration is usually proportional to the lipid solubility of the drug; an un-ionized drug is more lipid soluble than an ionized one. Inhaling drugs reduces but does not completely prevent systemic side effects.

D50 FTFFF
School refusal is due to an irrational fear of attending school. It commonly presents with abdominal pain, headaches or vague symptoms. In contrast to truants, the child is reluctant to leave home in the morning, is typically academically good and is a conformist at school. Approximately one-third continue with neurotic symptoms and social impairment in adult life.

D51 FTTTF
Respiratory syncytial virus (RSV) is the virus most commonly implicated in acute viral bronchiolitis, although it may also cause a range of other upper and lower respiratory tract infections. Clinical features of acute viral bronchiolitis include cough, tachypnoea, hyperinflation and recession with wheeze, occasional grunting, fine inspiratory and expiratory crackles and feeding difficulty. The illness is generally more severe in infants with pre-existing cardiopulmonary disease. Recurrent cough and wheeze are recognized complications and there is evidence that asthmatic symptoms are increased as much as 10 years later. There is a small group of infants in whom structural change at the time of the acute infection may lead to more severe chronic respiratory morbidity, and in whom there is a risk of bronchitis and emphysema in adult life.

D52 FFFFT
Identification of raised concentrations of sodium and chloride in the sweat is the principal diagnostic test for cystic fibrosis (CF). Short stature and pubertal delay are non-specific complications of chronic illness and are by no means inevitable in patients with CF, particularly in those with well controlled disease. Pathological abnormalities of the portal tracts and fatty infiltration are common but the spectrum of presentation of liver disease in cystic fibrosis is wide, ranging from prolonged jaundice in the newborn to cirrhosis and portal hypertension. The vast majority of males with CF are infertile due to maldevelopment of the vas deferens.

D53 FFFTT
There is typically an increase in residual volume and functional residual capacity in the asthmatic patient, because of air trapping.

The FEV_1 is reduced and the FEV_1/FVC ratio is therefore less than normal. The FVC is not expected to show a 20% increase following a bronchodilator, but the FEV_1 typically does. Asthma affects the medium and small airways, resulting in a decrease of the FEF_{25} and FEF_{75}. Asthma does not influence diffusion of gases across alveoli.

D54 TFTFF
Sudden infant death syndrome (SIDS) is most common between 2 and 6 months of age with a peak at 3 months. When comparing SIDS between countries and certain ethnic groups in a country, it is important to realize that different countries may have different extents to which a pathologist will pursue an alternative diagnosis and different communities will have differing social class structures, maternal ages and smoking habits. Having said this, it appears that there are genuine differences in SIDS rates; for example, rates are high in New Zealand, particularly among Maoris, but are low in Hong Kong. Asians have been shown to have a lower SIDS rate than whites in California and in England and Wales. The death rate is higher in social classes IV and V, where antenatal care has not been sought, when mothers smoke and where fathers are absent. Infants of low birthweight are at greater risk, whether due to prematurity, intrauterine growth retardation or multiple birth. SIDS is more common in second or subsequent babies than in first born infants.

D55 FTTFF
Projectile vomiting is the classical symptom of pyloric stenosis. Babies typically feed hungrily and vomit straight afterwards. During feeds, peristalsis may be visible over the stomach and a small mass may be palpable in the upper abdomen, usually just to the right of the midline – these findings are the basis of the test feed. The characteristic metabolic finding is hypochloraemic alkalosis.

D56 TTFTT
The chi square (X^2) test relates to the frequencies of occurrence, not on quantitative or qualitative data, and may therefore be used to determine whether the frequencies with which certain characteristics are found differ significantly from those expected under the null hypothesis or an alternative hypothesis. The degrees of freedom of a statistic are the number of unrestricted variables associated with it and therefore are one less than the number of variables in a X^2 table.

D57 TTTTT

Complications of diabetes mellitus are rare before puberty or in individuals with diabetes for less than 8–10 years. Diabetic nephropathy is associated with hypertension and proteinuria and may be detected early by careful monitoring of blood pressure and urine. Lipohypertrophy is manifest as lumpiness at injection sites and results from the local action of insulin, reflecting inadequate rotation of injection sites. Lipoatrophy results from immune responses to bovine insulin, appearing as dimples at injection sites and is rarely seen now that synthetic human or highly purified porcine insulins are in general use. Diabetes mellitus is associated with an increased incidence of coeliac disease, thyroid disease and other autoimmune disorders. Blood fructosamine levels reflect blood glucose over a period of about 3 weeks and may therefore be used to monitor glycaemic control as an alternative to, or alongside, glycosylated haemoglobin (HbA1C) which reflects levels over about 2 months.

D58 TTTFF

Craniopharyngiomas are histologically benign tumours of Rathke's pouch which may be cystic or solid,with or without calcification, and tend to erode surrounding structures. They cause hormonal disturbance in 80–90% of patients. They may present with raised intracranial pressure or visual field disturbances or with the consequences of hormonal deficiencies, in particular diabetes insipidus and short stature. Treatment of symptomatic tumours consists of surgery, with radiotherapy added for incompletely resected tumours. Chemotherapy has not been shown to be effective. About two-thirds of cases occur before the age of 20 and the median age of onset is 8 years. The prognosis is worse in children under the age of 5, in incompletely resected tumours and in those with a less cystic morphology. Recurrence rates are highest in the first 2 years after diagnosis and long-term morbidity is common.

D59 TTFTT

Nystagmus is usually due to a defect of vision such as optic atrophy or cataract. It almost always occurs in albinism, and is also associated with many drugs including anticonvulsants but not anticoagulants. Spasmus nutans is a disorder in which jerky head movements and nystagmus disappear when the child concentrates on an object. Diseases of the cerebellum or cerebellar tracts result in ataxia and nystagmus. Examples include Friedreich's ataxia, tumours or infections. Nystagmus may also follow an intraventricular haemorrhage in the newborn.

D60 TTFFF

Terbutaline and salbutamol are used to treat bronchoconstriction, but they may also cause a paradoxical bronchoconstriction. Non-steroidal anti-inflammatory drugs such as ibuprofen and diclofenac may worsen bronchospasm. High doses of morphine may also have a bronchoconstrictor effect.

Practice examination E   Answers

E1 TFTTF
The facial nerve supplies the muscles of the face, the cheek and scalp, the stylohyoid, the posterior belly of the digastric muscles of the neck and the stapedius muscle of the middle ear. The sensory root carries taste fibres from the anterior two-thirds of the tongue, the floor of the mouth and the soft palate. The parasympathetic fibres supply the submandibular and sublingual salivary glands, the lacrimal glands and the glands of the nose and palate. Lower motor neuron lesions (e.g. in the internal auditory meatus, the middle ear or parotid gland) cause weakness of the whole side of the face giving incomplete eye closure, loss of forehead wrinkling and the mouth sags on the affected side. An upper motor neuron lesion spares the upper part of the face because the neurons supplying this area receive fibres from both cerebral cortices. Lesions of the facial nerve proximal to the middle ear, where the chorda tympani leaves, cause loss of taste over the anterior two-thirds of the tongue. The facial skin receives its sensory supply from the three divisions of the trigeminal nerve. The lateral rectus is supplied by the abducent nerve.

E2 TFFTT
In pyloric stenosis, gastric acid and potassium are lost and, as a consequence, there is less chloride available for renal excretion. Bartter's syndrome is a disorder of renal tubular reabsorption of chloride, and therefore also sodium, leading to enhanced exchange of sodium with potassium and hydrogen ions in the distal tubule (secondary hyperaldosteronism). The result is hypochloraemic alkalosis, hypokalaemia, hyponatraemia and a high urinary chloride. Pseudo–Bartter's syndrome is seen in some children with cystic fibrosis and results from loss of sodium and chloride in the sweat. The metabolic picture is similar to that of Bartter's syndrome, but there is a low urinary chloride level. Congenital chloridorrhoea results from a defect in chloride and bicarbonate transport in the ileum and colon, leading to secondary hyperaldosteronism, and low urinary chloride.

E3 FTFTT
Magnesium is an important intracellular cation, acting as a coenzyme for many reactions and contributing to neuromuscular excitability. It is present in most foodstuffs, but its highest levels are found in cereals and green vegetables. Excretion is mainly renal, although there is some intestinal loss. Active reabsorption of magnesium takes place in the proximal convoluted tubule and loop of Henle, and is increased by hypomagnesaemia, hypocalcaemia

and parathyroid hormone. Magnesium excess rarely occurs in the absence of impaired renal function, but may follow excessive intake through medication and occasionally increased gut absorption due to hyperparathyroidism or hyperthyroidism. It may lead to hyporeflexia, respiratory depression, drowsiness and ultimately coma, but symptoms may be reversed rapidly by the administration of calcium infusions. Deficiency of magnesium is rarely due to problems of intake. In the newborn, hypomagnesaemia may mimic the symptoms of hypocalcaemia, with which it often coexists. Administration of calcium alone may make the symptoms worse, whereas magnesium supplementation may restore levels of both ions to normal.

E4 FFTTT
Approximately 55% of cardiac output passes through the placenta leaving only 45% to pass through the fetal tissues. Oxygenated blood passes from the umbilical vein to the ductus venosus, into the inferior vena cava and right atrium.

E5 TFFFT
Pulmonary stenosis is seen in patients with congenital rubella, Noonan syndrome, William's syndrome and tetralogy of Fallot. Turner syndrome has an association with left heart lesions with coarctation of the aorta occuring in approximately 10%. Holt Oram syndrome is associated with atrial septal defects and Friedreich's ataxia with cardiomyopathy.

E6 TFTTT
When pulmonary blood flow is increased, the main branches of the pulmonary artery are increased in size – pulmonary plethora. Causes of increased pulmonary blood flow include transposition of the great arteries, total anomalous pulmonary venous drainage, patent ductus arteriosus, ventricular septal defect, atrial septal defect and truncus arteriosus. If pulmonary blood flow is reduced, as in tetralogy of Fallot, critical pulmonary stenosis and severe Ebstein's anomaly, the lung fields are oligaemic.

E7 FFFTT
An infant may be cyanosed due to cardiac, respiratory or neurological causes. Transposition of the great arteries is the most common congenital cardiac defect presenting in the newborn infant. Some infants with cyanotic heart disease require a prostaglandin infusion to maintain the ductus and improve the hypoxia and metabolic acidosis while awaiting intervention. In

the hyperoxia test or nitrogen washout, where the Pa_{O_2} is measured from the right radial artery after 15 minutes of breathing 100% oxygen, cyanotic congenital heart disease is likely if the result is less than 20 kPa and extremely unlikely if the Pa_{O_2} is greater than 33 kPa. Indomethacin is used to close a patent ductus arteriosus and might be harmful in a cyanosed neonate. In total anomalous pulmonary venous drainage, the pulmonary veins drain into the right atrium either directly or indirectly. It usually presents with heart failure, although cyanosis may develop later as a result of raised right atrial pressure if the lesion is associated with atrial septal defect. Bacterial endocarditis is extremely rare in infancy.

E8 TTFFF
Scissoring is abnormal at any age. Hand preference is abnormal before the age of 15 months and therefore may indicate asymmetrical weakness. Median age for walking unaided is 13 months but many children take much longer, especially if bottom shufflers. Investigation, looking for muscular dystrophy in particular, would be recommended in a boy who fails to walk by 18 months. Approximately 10–15% of 5 year olds, 5% of 10 year olds and 1% of 15 year olds have nocturnal enuresis. Intervention is rarely considered before the age of 6 years. Most children have one or two words by the age of 1 year, but there is no cause for concern unless there are still no words by 18 months.

E9 FTFTF
The development of manipulative (fine motor) skills and vision are closely linked and therefore considered together. Infants can fix on their mother's face at around 3–4 weeks of age and will follow through 90° by 6 weeks, but following through 180° takes 3 months to develop. They will reach for objects using a palmar grasp between 4 and 5 months and with a crude pincer grasp from 9 to 10 months. Building towers of 2.5 cm bricks is a useful simple screen – at 18 months a child should manage three cubes, rising to at least 10 cubes by the age of four. Drawing skills start with a to and fro scribble at 18 months, circular scribble at 2, copying a circle at 3, a cross at 4 and a square and triangle at 5. The drawing of shapes in imitation of an adult can usually be achieved approximately 6 months before the ability to copy a completed shape. Strabismus (squint) is not uncommon in young infants who are learning to converge and fix on objects, but should be investigated if persistent at 6 months.

E10 TTFFT
The neural tube usually closes on day 27 post-conception. There are three primitive vesicles, the rhombencephalon, mesencephalon (midbrain) and prosencephalon (forebrain), which subdivides into diencephalon and telencephalon. The cerebellum, together with medulla and pons, develops from the rhombencephalon and the telencephalon gives rise to the cerebral hemispheres. Sensory neurons are contained in the alar plate, and motor neurons in the basal plate of the spinal cord.

E11 FFTFT
A patient with carbon monoxide poisoning is typically pink but has symptoms of hypoxia which include confusion, headache and coma. Carbon monoxide binds to haemoglobin at the same point as oxygen but this bond is approximately 230 times stronger. The arterial Po_2 remains normal despite the reduced oxyhaemoglobin and chemoreceptors that increase respiratory drive therefore remain unstimulated. The carboxyhaemoglobin concentration remains static if ventilation ceases allowing confirmation of the diagnosis for a long time after death. The only treatment is administration of a high enough Po_2 to displace the carboxyhaemoglobin. This may necessitate the use of hyperbaric oxygen.

E12 TFFFT
If the sex is not immediately obvious, far less emotional trauma is likely to result if it is honestly stated that further assessment and investigations are required to establish the sex, than if the incorrect sex is assigned confidently in the delivery room. Karyotype is not the only determinant of sex of rearing as it is vital to consider functional aspects: there is little point in attempting to raise a child with a 46XY karyotype as a boy, if he has no prospect of being able to pass urine standing up or achieve a useful erection. All cases should be regarded as potential cases of salt-losing congenital adrenal hyperplasia, until proved otherwise, because of the disastrous consequences of missing the condition. Clitoral reduction and vaginoplasty may be performed as early as 2 months of age. There is a high risk of malignancy developing in dysgenetic gonads, so removal should be regarded as a relative emergency.

E13 FTFFF
Hypoglycaemia is commonly seen in infants of diabetics as they are hyperinsulinaemic. Growth hormone deficiency may present with hypoglycaemia in infancy before there is any recognizable

effect on stature. Ketonuria does not occur in the presence of
adequate insulin levels. In diabetics, ketonuria is seen in association with raised blood glucose and hypoglycaemia occurs following insulin overdose, after excessive exercise, or after missing a
meal. Infant brains are very susceptible to hypoglycaemic damage
whereas older children and adults are more resilient. Slow correction with an infusion of 10% dextrose is adequate and is far less
likely to lead to rebound hypoglycaemia or potentially dangerous
osmotic changes, resulting from overdosage.

E14 FFFFT
People with diabetes should eat a diet similar to a healthy diet of
a non-diabetic. The proportion of carbohydrate should be enough
to allow a reasonably low fat intake, and is best eaten in the form
of starchy high fibre foods. Rapidly absorbed sugary foods do not
allow good glycaemic control and should be avoided. Exercise
should be encouraged as it improves general fitness and is important for social and psychological reasons. Strenuous exercise may
cause problems with glycaemic control but many patients manage
to adapt their carbohydrate intake and insulin dose to suit the
intensity of exercise planned. It is sensible to have additional
snacks available. Insulin is needed even if there is no dietary
intake due to illness, and requirements are often increased. Blood
glucose estimations should be monitored throughout the illness.
The rate of insulin absorption varies with exercise, if the site is
rubbed after injection and if there is lipohypertrophy due to
repeated use of the same injection site.

E15 FFTTF
ADH is responsible for conserving body water and regulating the
osmolarity of body fluids. Factors that stimulate secretion include
a decrease in blood volume, an increased plasma osmolarity, pain,
hypotension, stress and hyperthermia. Its secretion is inhibited by
decreased plasma osmolarity, alcohol, α-adrenergic agonists,
cortisol and hypothermia.

E16 TTFTT
Hirschsprung's disease should be suspected if there has been
delay in the passage of meconium beyond the first 24 h of life. All
opiates have the tendency to constipate. Poor fluid intake, a diet
low in fibre and/or high in dairy products may all lead to constipation. Predisposing medical conditions include hypercalcaemia
and other causes of polyuria, hypothyroidism, coeliac disease,
cow's milk protein intolerance and lead poisoning. Any form of

emotional disturbance may lead to constipation. More specifically, penetrative anal abuse may result in anal pain and consequent reluctance to defaecate.

E17 FTTFT
The bile salts, cholate and chenodesoxycholate, are formed in the liver from cholesterol. They are conjugated with taurine, glycine and ornithine and secreted in the bile. Bile salts in the intestinal tract emulsify fat globules and also aid absorption of fatty acids and other lipids by complexing with them to form micelles which are highly soluble. Bile salts are essential for the satisfactory absorption of fat-soluble vitamins (A, D, E and K). Approximately 94% of bile salts are reabsorbed by active transport in the distal ileum. They pass by the portal blood to the liver and are recirculated into the bile.

E18 FFTFT
Alpha-1-antitrypsin (α-1-AT) is a protease inhibitor that controls various inflammatory cascades. Deficiency is associated with liver disease and pulmonary emphysema, especially in smokers. The genetic variants are described by their electrophoretic mobilities as medium (M), slow (S) or very slow (Z). The normal genotype is PiMM. Patients who are homozygotes for the Z allele (PiZZ) have low α-1-AT and are usually severely affected by liver disease. Heterozygotes (e.g. PiMZ) have a variable phenotype and may develop signs of deficiency. Currently there is no specific therapy available.

E19 FTFTF
Macroglossia occurs in hypothyroidism, Beckwith–Wiedemann syndrome and glycogen storage disease type II. The tongue appears big in Down's syndrome because of the relatively small mouth and because hypotonia causes it to protrude. It is smooth in familial dysautonomia because of the absence of papillae. In scarlet fever the tongue initially appears swollen with a white coating. As the coating disappears it takes on the red 'strawberry' appearance.

E20 FFTTF
Coeliac disease has not been identified as a single gene disorder, although the increased incidence in first degree relatives and association with HLA-B8 emphasize the importance of genetic factors. Blood groups A and B show codominance as both traits are expressed in the heterozygote. Periodic paralysis exists in both autosomal dominant and recessive forms. 11β-Hydroxylase

deficiency, the second most common cause of congenital adrenal hyperplasia, is autosomal recessive.

E21 FFFTT

The Barr body, also known as the sex chromatin, consists of one condensed X chromosome, found within the nucleus of somatic cells with more than one X chromosome. In general, the number of Barr bodies is one less than the number of X chromosomes. Turner syndrome is associated with a 45X karyotype, complete androgen insensitivity syndrome with XY and Klinefelter syndrome with XXY. Oocytes are haploid and therefore only contain one X chromosome.

E22 TTFFF

Fragile X is the most common cause of mental retardation in males after Down's syndrome, with an incidence of 1 per 1000 males. The key features are mental retardation, enlarged testes following puberty and an X chromosome fragile site. The facial phenotype becomes more obvious in older children – a large forehead, long nose, prominent chin and big ears. Female distribution of secondary sexual hair is associated with Klinefelter syndrome. Up to 30% of carrier females have developmental delay which is usually mild, but may be as severe as affected males.

E23 FTTTF

Neonatal alloimmune thrombocytopenia (NAIT) is the platelet counterpart of haemolytic disease of the newborn. The infant inherits a platelet antigen from the father, which is lacking in the mother. There may be manifestations as early as 14 weeks' gestation, as soon as maternal antibodies against the fetal platelets cross the placenta. Antenatal treatment is controversial; a single tranfusion of PlA1 negative (or washed maternal) platelets may protect against the dangers of traumatic delivery, but will not influence the outcome where there has been earlier bleeding. Frequent antenatal transfusions are required for adequate cover. Immunoglobulins and steroids have also been employed.

E24 TFTFF

Jaundice, pallor and splenomegaly are recognized clinical features of haemolysis. The reticulocyte count is raised and haptoglobin levels depressed due to saturation with haemoglobin. In extravascular haemolysis, red cell destruction takes place in the reticuloendothelial system. Haemoglobinuria is seen only in cases of intravascular haemolysis.

E25 FTFTF
In early embryonic life primitive red cell production takes place in the yolk sac. By the second trimester the liver is the main site of production with some also produced in the spleen and lymph nodes. In later pregnancy and after birth, red cells are produced exclusively by the bone marrow. The bone marrow of the long bones becomes increasingly fatty from 5 years of age and under normal circumstances stops red cell production from approximately 20 years of age, when production is confined to the membranous bones (vertebrae, ribs and pelvis). There is no direct response of the bone marrow to hypoxia. Hypoxia stimulates erythropoietin production almost immediately but the red cell response in the circulation is not seen for some days. Maturation of the red cell is dependent on vitamin B_{12} and folic acid.

E26 TTTTT
Local and systemic effects of mast cell disorders are attributed to the release of histamine, leukotrienes, heparin and proteases. The spectrum of disease includes urticaria pigmentosa, caused by large collections of mast cells in 'nests' within the dermis, seen mainly in infancy and usually self limiting. Generalized itching and flushing is sometimes associated with the rash, and variants include blisters rather than the lightly pigmented swellings of classic urticaria pigmentosa. Systemic mastocytosis is a more severe manifestation, seen mainly in adults. It is characterized by infiltration of organs including liver, spleen, bone marrow, bone and skin. The most malignant form may culminate in mast cell leukaemia.

E27 FTTFT
The presence of opsonins on the surface of bacteria facilitates phagocytosis. The most important opsonic factors are IgG and complement (C3). Other opsonins include acute phase reactants such as C reactive protein. IgD is a surface molecule on the membrane of B cells and has a role in regulating the differentiation and maturation of these cells.

E28 TTFFT
Ataxia telangiectasia is associated with a combined immunodeficiency which predominantly leads to IgG deficiency. T cell defects also occur but are rarely complicated by opportunistic infections. Wiskott–Aldrich syndrome is an X-linked condition associated with thrombocytopenia, eczema and T cell lymphopenia. Bacterial infections are common and there may be infections with opportunistic pathogens. DiGeorge syndrome comprises absent thymus,

cell-mediated immunodeficiency, hypocalcaemia, congenital heart defects and characteristic facies. Schwachmann's sydrome is associated with a neutrophil chemotactic defect and chronic granulomatous disease is a disorder of neutrophil function.

E29 FTFTT
Glandular fever, or infectious mononucleosis, is caused by the Epstein Barr virus (EBV), but unlike other members of the herpes family of viruses, of which it is one, it does not cause ulceration as part of its clinical spectrum. Complications may involve practically any system and include airway obstruction, myocarditis, pneumonitis, orchitis, hepatitis, splenic rupture, haemolytic anaemia, thrombocytopenia, aplastic anaemia and neurological manifestations, ranging from cranial nerve palsies to Guillain–Barré syndrome. Renal manifestations are rare but an acute post-infectious glomerulonephritis has been described following infection with EBV, ECHO, coxsackie and influenza viruses.

E30 TTFFT
Brucellosis, or undulant fever, is caused by *Brucella abortus*, *melitensis* or *suis* and may exist as asymptomatic infection, acute brucellosis or chronic infection. It is most commonly transmitted to humans via infected milk but also by direct contact and through the skin. It often presents as a pyrexia of unknown origin and mainly affects the reticuloendothelial system, although osteomyelitis, arthritis, meningitis, encephalitis, peritonitis and endocarditis are all recognized complications. The organisms are difficult to grow in blood and the diagnosis is therefore primarily serological. Brucella is an intracellular pathogen and therefore frequently leads to a lymphocytosis with neutropenia.

E31 TTTFT
Erythema infectiosum is caused by human parvovirus B19 with epidemics classically occurring in winter and spring. It is said to mimic closely rubella. The first sign of infection is usually marked erythema of the cheeks (slapped cheek disease) with circumoral pallor. An itchy, erythematous rash later develops over the trunk and limbs, and this may fluctuate for several weeks. Malaise, mild pyrexia, myalgia and arthralgia or arthritis are other features of infection. Infection during pregnancy can result in hydrops fetalis but no anatomical abnormalities have been described in babies of infected mothers.

E32 FFTTF
Malaria is usually transmitted by the female *Anopheles* mosquito, but it may also be transferred by blood products or transplacentally. Enlargement of the spleen and liver is common in acute and chronic infections. The illness may be complicated by cerebral malaria and profound anaemia. Other complications which are less common in children include renal failure, pulmonary oedema and disseminated intravascular coagulation. The presence of haemoglobin S, glucose-6-phosphatase deficiency, thalassaemia and pyridoxal kinase deficiency offer some resistance against falciparum malaria. The fever of falciparum malaria is often irregular, but if a pattern is evident the spikes of temperature are at less than 48 h intervals.

E33 TTFFF
Polyarticular onset juvenile chronic arthritis (JCA) involves five or more joints, usually symmetrically. It may be classified by the presence or absence of IgM rheumatoid factor, those who are positive being more likely to have destructive disease that responds poorly to drug therapy. The commonest joints involved are the knees, wrists, ankles, hips and small joints of the hands with sparing of the metacarpophalangeal joints. Involvement of the cervical spine and temporomandibular joints also occurs fairly commonly. Iridocyclitis occurs occasionally in patients with polyarthritis but the incidence is much higher in those with pauciarticular onset JCA.

E34 FFFFT
Surfactant is a lipidoprotein, also known as dipalmitoyl phosphatidylcholine, synthesized by the type II alveolar epithelial cells, or granular pneumocytes. It reduces the surface tension in alveolae, thus preventing their collapse, and its deficiency in premature infants is a major cause of neonatal morbidity and mortality. Storage of surfactant is identifiable in type II cells at 24 weeks' gestation and delivery onto the alveolar surface can be detected from about 30 weeks onwards. Its production is impaired by acidosis, hypoxia and hypothermia. Treatment includes general supportive measures, such as supplementary oxygen and positive pressure ventilation, prophylaxis with maternal steroids and more specific treatment with natural or synthetic surfactant preparations, delivered via the endotracheal tube.

E35 TFTFT
Metabolic causes of neonatal seizures include hypoglycaemia, hypocalcaemia, hypomagnesaemia, sodium and water imbalance

and a number of inborn errors of metabolism, such as the urea cycle disorders and amino acidaemias. Pyridoxine dependency is a rare autosomal recessive disorder which leads to seizures which are resistant to conventional anticonvulsants and sometimes associated with reports of increased fetal movements. Intracranial haemorrhage may be associated with seizures but isolated cephalhaematoma, if severe enough to produce systemic complications, leads only to anaemia and jaundice. Intracranial infections are common causes of neonatal seizures, whether bacterial, usually secondary to group B streptococcal or *E. coli* infection, viral, due to infection with herpes simplex, rubella, cytomegalovirus or coxsackie B, or secondary to toxoplasmosis. Other causes include hypoxic-ischaemic encephalopathy, abnormalities of brain development, narcotic withdrawal, toxins, autosomal dominant familial neonatal seizures and the benign 'fifth day fits'.

E36 TTTTT
Necrotizing enterocolitis (NEC) is a neonatal disease of unknown aetiology. It is usually sporadic but epidemic outbreaks in neonatal units are not uncommon. Presenting features inlude bile stained aspirates, vomiting, bloody diarrhoea and a tender, distended abdomen, but the infant may present with a non-specific collapse. Complications include septic shock, metabolic acidosis, disseminated intravascular coagulation, bowel perforation, late stenosis and malabsorption during the recovery phase. Investigation should include a plain X-ray which may show distended loops of bowel, pneumatosis intestinalis, portal vein gas, pneumoperitoneum and free fluid levels. A full blood count may reveal thrombocytopenia and a neutrophilia or neutropenia with toxic granulations. Treatment is generally conservative, with parenteral feeding and antibiotics. The prognosis is improved by early identification of the condition but remains poor if complications requiring surgery develop.

E37 FTTTT
Pulmonary hypoplasia is present in 15% of neonatal deaths and occurs as a primary lesion in about 10% of cases. Lung hypoplasia may be caused by oligohydramnios from renal agenesis, bladder neck obstruction or prolonged rupture of membranes. It may also result from thoracic space occupying lesions such as diaphragmatic hernia, pleural effusions or cysts. Normal fetal lung growth is dependent upon fetal breathing and any lack of such lung movement can result in hypoplasia. Neurological anomalies (e.g. anencephaly), congenital muscular disorders, absent diaphragm and exomphalos all prevent normal fetal breathing.

E38 FFFTT
Increased glomerular permeability results from decreased negative charge. In both benign postural proteinuria and many of the pathological causes of proteinuria, protein excretion increases as the day progresses. Microalbuminuria is a marker of early diabetic nephropathy. Wilson's disease may cause a proximal renal tubular acidosis, with impaired reabsorption of glucose, bicarbonate, phosphate and amino acids. Timed urine collections are technically difficult in children. Measurement of protein:creatinine ratios in single voided urine samples has a high correlation with 24-h urine excretion rates, although individual clinicians vary in their readiness to accept this evidence without proceeding to timed collections.

E39 TFFFT
Vesicoureteric reflux may lead to renal impairment and the kidneys may be enlarged secondary to hydronephrosis, normal in size or shrunk due to scarring. Minimal change nephrotic syndrome does not cause impairment of renal excretory function and the kidneys are likely to be normal in size or slightly oedematous. Wilms' tumour leads to massive enlargement of the affected kidney(s) and impaired renal function is unusual at presentation.

E40 FTFFT
The normal EEG in childhood shows immature features, including slow (θ and δ) rhythms with frontal and temporal predominance which disappear in adult life as the EEG matures. Hypsarrhythmia is the characteristic feature of infantile spasms, the causes of which are multiple and include cerebral malformations, congenital infections and metabolic disorders. A generalized pattern of slow waves is suggestive of an infective or metabolic encephalopathy, whereas an abscess is likely to produce a focal pattern. A 3 Hz spike and wave pattern is seen in primary generalized, or petit mal, epilepsy which is not associated with structural brain abnormalities. Burst suppression is seen in cases of severe brain injury, including subacute sclerosing panencephalitis.

E41 TFFFT
Cerebral blood flow represents 15% of cardiac output despite the brain representing only 2% of the adult mass. Elevated CO_2 increases cerebral blood flow as does hypoxia. Sympathetic and parasympathetic nerves have little or no effect on cerebral vessels. Cerebral blood flow is autoregulated so that changes in blood pressure within the normal range have no significant influence.

E42 TFFFT
Vitamin A deficiency is associated with ocular defects (xeroph-thalmia) and an increased susceptibility to infections. Deficiency in the UK is rare even in disorders of fat absorption. Children under the care of a cystic fibrosis clinic will be on pancreatic enzyme supplements and vitamin A supplements making clinical deficiency extremely unlikely. Healthy women who are planning conception or who are pregnant are advised not to take vitamin A supplements as high levels of the vitamin may lead to birth defects.

E43 TTFTF
Wilms' tumours (nephroblastomas) occur in 1 in 10 000 live births with no sex predominance and a peak age of 3 years. Up to 20% of unilateral tumours and almost all bilateral tumours are inher-ited. Associations with Wilms' tumour include aniridia, hemihy-pertrophy and genitourinary anomalies. Infants with Beckwith–Wiedemann syndrome may have persistent hypogly-caemia, exomphalos, macroglossia, visceromegaly and parallel creases on the ear lobes. It is associated with Wilms' tumour and hepatoblastoma.

E44 FFTTF
A bitemporal hemianopia results from central compression of the optic chiasm, affecting the decussation of nasal fibres of the optic nerves. The commonest cause is a tumour of the pituitary, but a similar field defect may be caused by a craniopharyngioma, suprasellar meningioma or carotid aneurysm and rarely cerebrovascular accident or trauma.

E45 TTFFT
Maternal narcotic use leads to the most severe reactions but symptoms are also seen with alcohol, barbiturates, benzodi-azepines, chlorpromazine, glutethimide, lithium, and tricyclic antidepressants.

E46 FTTTT
Nitric oxide (NO) has been identified as endothelium derived relaxing factor (EDRF) which is produced by endothelial cells in response to acetylcholine. Nitric oxide synthase catalyses the synthesis of NO from the amino acid arginine. Its action is very short lived as it is rapidly oxidized to nitrogen dioxide, nitrite and nitrate and inactivated in the blood by binding to haemoglobin. NO is a very potent vasodilator and also has some activity as a

bronchodilator, a non-cholinergic, non-adrenergic neurotransmitter and as an inflammatory mediator. Its clinical applications as an inhaled therapy exploit its qualities as a pulmonary vasodilator in conditions characterized by pulmonary vasoconstriction and ventilation perfusion mismatch. It has been found to be of benefit in infants with pulmonary hypertension secondary to congential heart disease, persistent fetal circulation, respiratory distress syndrome and bronchopulmonary dysplasia and in older patients with respiratory failure due to adult respiratory distress syndrome.

E47 TTTTF

Calcium resonium and sodium polystyrene sulphonate are ion-exchange resins which can be used in the treatment of hyperkalaemia. These oral preparations are unabsorbed and exchange potassium for calcium or sodium ions. The potassium is thereby removed at a greater rate than that at which it is entering the extracellular fluid. Plasma potassium can be rapidly reduced by an infusion of glucose and insulin, the insulin increasing the rate of entry of potassium into cells. Severe hyperkalaemia can cause cardiac arrest but the affect on the myocardium may be reduced by the opposing action of calcium as a sodium gluconate infusion while waiting for other treatments to reduce the serum potassium level. Salbutamol lowers serum potassium, and when used in large doses for the treatment of acute asthma, the serum potassium should be monitored to avoid dangerous hypokalaemia.

E48 TTFTT

Side effects of the β-antagonists depend to some extent on their selectivity. Cardiac effects include slowing of conduction through the atrioventricular node, antidysrhythmic effects, negative inotropic and chronotropic effects, decreased left ventricular ejection secondary to peripheral vasoconstriction and precipitation of cardiac failure, particularly in patients who were previously compensated. Non-selective β-blockers cause bronchoconstriction. β-Antagonists interfere with glycogenolysis and may exacerbate hypoglycaemia. They cross the blood–brain barrier causing fatigue, memory loss and occasionally psychotic reactions. They also cross the placenta causing bradycardia, hypotension and hypoglycaemia in the newborn infants of mothers who are on medication.

E49 TFFFF

Warfarin is a synthetic coumarin which prevents the synthesis of vitamin K dependent clotting factors (II, VII, IX and X) in the liver. Haemorrhage is the most common side effect and gastrointestinal upsets may occur. The drug is teratogenic if taken during the first trimester of pregnancy. The activity of warfarin may be potentiated by alcohol, cimetidine, salicylates and many antibiotics which inhibit hepatic metabolism. Its activity is decreased by drugs which induce hepatic enzymes including barbiturates, the oral contraceptive pill and carbamezepine. Acute reversal of warfarin's effects can be achieved by administration of fresh frozen plasma. Vitamin K reverses its effects within 12 h.

E50 TTFTF
Schizophrenia is rare in adolescents and at least 10% have a positive family history. There are no specific childhood precursors of the disease. Its onset is often insidious and first rank symptoms may not be present in the early stages. Neuroleptic drugs are the treatment of choice.

E51 FTFFF
Inhaled treatment for asthma is best delivered by metered dose inhaler via a spacer device in very young children. However, the use of spacers for delivery of inhaled steroids is often recommended in older children because of improved efficiency of drug delivery, reduced oral deposition and reduced systemic absorption. From the age of 4–6 years, most children can manage an inhaled powder device and, from 10, a metered dose inhaler without a spacer. Sodium cromoglycate is generally used in milder cases requiring prophylaxis, as compared to inhaled steroids, although some prescribers use low-dose steroids as a first line treatment and, conversely, cromoglycate may, on occasions, be effective in more severe cases. There is some concern about the effects of high-dose inhaled steroids on growth and adrenal suppression, but low-dose treatment has not been shown to have a significant measurable effect on growth. Peak flow measurements are useful for monitoring children of 5 years and over, but are rarely reliable in younger children.

E52 TFTTT
Bronchiectasis means dilatation of the bronchi. The bronchial walls become inflamed and thickened and the disease is characterized by cough productive of large amounts of purulent sputum. Bronchiectasis now mainly has its origins in childhood, either as a result of cystic fibrosis or other congenital bronchial abnormalities, including Williams–Campbell syndrome and ciliary dyskinesia, part of Kartagener's syndrome. It is now a very unusual

complication of whooping cough, measles and bacterial pneumonia in the developed world, but may be acquired as a consequence of aspiration of a foreign body which has gone unnoticed, post primary tuberculosis and chronic chest infection in the presence of immune deficiency.

E53 FTTFT

The administration of 100% oxygen leads to a slight decrease in the heart rate and a decrease of 8–20% in cardiac output. The pulmonary vascular resistance and mean pulmonary artery pressure decrease. Nitrogen is eliminated from the lungs within 2 minutes leading to atelectasis because of the loss of the 'splinting' effect of nitrogen. Oxygen administration has no effect on glucose utilization.

E54 TTTTT

Most lung disease is associated with an increased risk of pneumothorax, although in most conditions this risk remains fairly small. In addition to primary respiratory diseases, pneumothorax may occur in collagen disorders such as Ehlers–Danlos and Marfan's syndromes, and in association with mechanical ventilation.

E55 TTTTF

There are numerous causes of neck stiffness in childhood ranging from trivial viral infections to life-threatening meningitis. Meningism occurs in infections of the central nervous system such as poliomyelitis and encephalitis. It may also occur in many other childhood infections including mumps, tonsillitis, pneumonia and any illness causing cervical lymphadenopathy. Intracranial causes include haemorrhage, abscesses and tumours. Rheumatological diseases may cause neck stiffness with or without pain. Fibrodysplasia ossificans is a progressive disease in which the fibrous tissue of ligaments, aponeuroses and muscles become oedematous with areas of calcification and ectopic bone formation. It usually commences in the neck and back.

E56 TFFFT

The normal distribution is unimodal and symmetrical and the mean, mode and median are all the same value. It is a continuous probability distribution characterized by two parameters, the mean and variance, which fully describe the distribution; 68% of the observations are within one standard deviation of the mean and 95% within two standard deviations. The binomial and

Poisson distributions, which are both discrete probability distributions, may be approximated by the normal distribution as the number of events increases.

E57 TTFFT
The majority of cases of secondary hypertension in childhood are caused by renal parenchymal disease, of which reflux nephropathy is the most common. Vascular causes include renal artery abnormalities and renal vein thrombosis as well as coarctation of the aorta. Endocrine causes are uncommon in childhood but include adrenal hyperplasia and adenomata, phaeochromocytoma, neuroblastoma and Cushing's syndrome, most likely to be due to corticosteroid therapy. Among other causes of hypertension are intracranial tumours, lead poisoning, acute porphyria and drugs, but not diazoxide which is a potent antihypertensive for intravenous use.

E58 TTFFF
There are many different causes of the floppy infant. Those that are floppy and strong are likely to have central nervous system (upper motor neuron) or non-neurological causes. Diplegic cerebral palsy may be manifest as hypotonia, dystonia or spasticity. Floppy and weak infants have peripheral neuromuscular disease which may be subdivided according to the part of the neuromuscular apparatus affected. Werdnig–Hoffman syndrome, or spinal muscular atrophy type 1, is an example of anterior horn cell disease. Peripheral neuropathies include Guillain–Barré syndrome, rarely affecting infants, and peroneal muscular atrophy, or Charcot–Marie–Tooth disease, which produces distal weakness and also rarely presents in infancy. Disorders affecting the neuromuscular junction include myasthenia gravis which presents later in childhood and rarely with generalized weakness or hypotonia, and neonatal myasthenia, a transient condition seen in about 15% of infants of myasthenic mothers; such infants may be floppy but symptoms resolve by 4–6 weeks. Muscle disorders leading to generalized hypotonia at 3 months include the congenital myopathies and congenital muscular dystrophy, but not Duchenne muscular dystrophy which usually presents between 1 and 4 years of age.

E59 TFTFF
Obsessive compulsive disorders are characterized by the compulsion to carry out some action, to recall an experience or thought or to ruminate on an abstract topic. Obsessional actions may be

ritualistic performances designed to relieve anxiety such as hand washing to cope with contamination. The patient recognizes his symptoms as absurd and this leads to anxiety and distress. Passivity feelings are when the subject believes that his thoughts, emotions or actions are controlled by an outside agency and are a feature of schizophrenia. Hallucinations may occur in the functional psychoses and in organic states, but are not a feature of neuroses.

E60 FTTFT
Maternal phenylketonuria (PKU) causes a risk to the fetus of spontaneous abortion, mental retardation, microcephaly, congenital heart disease and low birthweight. These risks increase with higher blood levels of phenylalanine. A restricted diet should be started before conception – the outcome is not so good if started after conception. Blood levels should be closely monitored and the diet intensively supervised as nutritional excesses or deficiencies may occur which are harmful to the fetus. Cord blood levels of phenylalanine are not elevated in PKU as the baby's levels only start to rise within the first day or so. Children born to mothers with high blood phenylalanine will have high cord blood levels which will drop rapidly after birth. PKU is an autosomal recessive disorder and the baby will not have the disease unless the father is affected or is a carrier.

Index